stories matter

stories matter

THE ROLE OF NARRATIVE IN MEDICAL ETHICS

EDITED BY

RITA CHARON & MARTHA MONTELLO

ROUTLEDGE

NEW YORK LONDON

Published in 2002 by
Routledge
29 West 35th Street
New York, NY 10001

Published in Great Britian by
Routledge
11 New Fetter Lane
London EC4P 4EE

Routledge is an imprint of the Taylor & Francis Group.

10 9 8 7 6 5 4 3 2 1

Library of Congress Cataloging-in-Publication Data

Stories matter : the role of narrative in medical ethics / edited by Rita Charon and Martha M. Montello.
     p. cm.—(Reflective bioethics)
Includes bibliographical references and index.
ISBN 0-415-92837-0 (hbk.) — ISBN 0-415-92838-9 (pbk.)
    1. Medical ethics. 2. Bioethics. 3. Narration (Rhetoric)—Psychological aspects. I. Charon, Rita. II. Montello, Martha M., 1949- III. Series.

R725.5 .S763 2002
174'.2—dc21   2001058180

CONTENTS

ACKNOWLEDGMENTS

We wish to acknowledge our deep and fortifying gratitude to our community of collegues in bioethics and in literary studies who have discovered, developed, and animated this youthful and hardy field of narrative ethics. In conferences, writing projects, teaching efforts, and research studies over the years, our colleagues have allowed us to trust in our early leanings toward a narrative practice of bioethics. We wish to acknowledge particularly the Society for Health and Human Values—now recently a part of the American Society for Bioethics and Humanities—as the incubator for much of this transdisciplinary thinking. Recent ASBH presidents Laurie Zoloth and Kathryn Montgomery have continued the fertile crossings between philosophy and literary studies that make our work possible.

This book project was initiated when Professor Stuart Spicker approached us to edit a special issue of *Healthcare Ethics Committee Forum* on narrative ethics, and we want to thank him for the idea. A parent of this book, the *HEC Forum* special issue helped to mobilize interest and commitment from many of our authors.

We'd like to recognize our own small band of literary collaborators who have been meeting and talking since the early 1980s as the Kaiser Narrative-in-Medicine Circle—Joanne Trautmann Banks, Julia E. Connelly, Anne Hunsaker Hawkins, Kathryn Montgomery, Anne Hudson Jones, and Suzanne Poirier—for decades of inspiration, challenge, education, and support.

Of course, we thank especially the twenty-two authors of this book's chapters for their knowledge, courage, vision, and eloquence. Our task as editors was merely a convening one; the authors poured forth their own convictions, cautions, and dreams. We are convinced that the world of bioethics will change by virtue of their work, and we feel humble in the face of what they have accomplished at our invitation.

The practical aspects of this book could not have been accomplished without the early passionate support of Hilde Lindemann Nelson and the efforts of Routledge editors Heidi Freund and Ilene Kalish. Assistant Editor Kimberly Guinta has been tremendously helpful and supportive along the way. We extend deep thanks to Benjamin Dov Frede for his meticulous editorial researching to confirm the accuracy of endnotes and textual citations—Dov's commitment to this book and his joy in working on it became a stabilizing and nourishing foundation for our own ongoing devotion to the work.

Rita wants to thank her husband, Bernard Gross, for his patience and generosity in making room for the book all this time. None of this work would matter without on-going lives of love and meaning. Martha wishes to thank her children, Anna and Paul, for their encouragement and abiding ability to keep life in perspective.

INTRODUCTION

MEMORY AND ANTICIPATION:
THE PRACTICE OF NARRATIVE ETHICS
RITA CHARON AND MARTHA MONTELLO

The practice of narrative ethics has developed organically, over the past two decades or so, germinating throughout North America, the United Kingdom, Europe, and parts of Asia, suggesting that this approach to ethics has answered a widespread need within the field. Not a top-down activity, narrative ethics emerged from individuals' ethics practices as they, often on their own, found themselves listening in new ways to their patients and thinking in new ways about cases. The public life of narrative ethics—this book, for example—is but a distal part of this process: nurses, doctors, ethicists, and patients have already made local discoveries that health care's primary duties are to bear witness to patients' suffering and to honor their experiences of illness. From those activities—if pursued with rigor, honesty, humility, and accuracy—flow choices, decisions, and actions. From them also flow healing dividends for patients and for caregivers.

Narrative ethics arose as doctors, nurses, ethicists, and patients found themselves taking seriously their acts of reading, writing, and telling. From patients' pathographies and caregivers' stories from practice to ethicists' written cases, what unified these early efforts was the recognition of the centrality of narrative in the work of health care. Although illness is, indeed, a biological and material phenomenon, the human response to it is neither biologically determined nor arithmetical. In extending help to a sick person, one not only determines what the matter might be; one also by the necessity of illness determines what its meanings might be. Such a search requires the narrative competence to follow the patient's narrative thread, to make sense of his or her figural language, to grasp the significance of stories told, and to imagine the illness from its conflicting perspectives. Narrative approaches to ethics recognize that the singular case emerges only in the act of narrating it and that duties are incurred in the act of hearing it. How the patient tells of illness, how the doctor or ethicist represents it in words, who listens as the intern presents at rounds, what the audience is being moved to feel or think—all these narrative dimensions of health care are of profound and defining importance in ethics and patient care.

Responding to a widespread narrativist turn of the time, bioethics is one of many fields of knowledge and practice to have been profoundly influenced by narrative theory. Various intellectual disciplines in the past two decades have taken the so-called narrativist turn: recognizing the extent to which perceptions are embedded in their telling, realizing human beings' reliance on storytelling to get their bearings in life, and acknowledging the innately narrative structure of human knowledge and provisional truth.[1] Historians, cognitive psychologists, social scientists, theologians, psychiatrists, and literary critics have come to recognize the central role that narrative plays in the way we construct knowledge, interpret experience, and define the right and the good.

The goal of this book is to guide readers toward a cognitive, practical, emotional, and aesthetic familiarity with the conceptual frameworks, methods, and powers of narrative ethics. The book's message—like narrative, its topic—unfolds in time. Readers will not find a statement of the propositions of narrative ethics. Nor will they find sets of rules or "steps" for its practice. Instead, like all narratives, this book conveys what truth it knows through a constant interplay among form, content, and the experiences incurred in reading it. We bring you thoughts and experiences of individuals in singular conversations and situations, not as precepts to be obeyed but as layers of exemplars to be absorbed. The experiences of individual authors—especially in the cases in part 3—will illuminate, we hope, the ways in which narrative practices, informed by the conceptual frameworks in parts 1 and 2, contribute to comprehending the ethical plights of patients, students, and professionals, guiding us all to recognize and perform fitting actions in the face of life.

All the authors of the essays ascribe to beliefs about human singularity, about the relational source of identity, and about language's unique power to define, describe, and expose what human beings see and can know. The writers gathered here from a range of intellectual disciplines, health fields, and stages in their own professional development suggest the wide range of the community we hope to engage in this textual conversation. A psychiatrist, a general internist, a pediatrician, an eminent literary critic, and a cognitive psychologist of international renown in the field of narrative knowledge are among the writers here who variously enter into dialogue about narrative approaches to ethics, observing and revealing the conceptual grounds upon which they do their work. The cases the clinicians bring under an ethical gaze consider the meanings of patients' lives over time, reflect on how those meanings change during the course of illness, and explore the way these changes in meaning give rise to the ethical questions at the heart of each narrative.

At the center of each case described in these chapters lies the recognition that serious illness raises the veil in the lives of those involved. Old family secrets, long-time troubling issues, deeply felt but unexpressed emotions—all muted or somehow removed from the surface of daily lives over the years—often become visible and expressed in ways that they are at no other time during our lives. Serious illness can be, and often is, a time of profound change in the lives of patients and those closest to them. What our authors understand and reveal is that narrative methods are uniquely capable of capturing, rendering, and conveying what these times are like for people for whom the veil has been lifted and how that reality affects the ways they perceive the moral choices open to them. And with the honed skill of good narrativists, all our writers show that arriving at a fitting resolution in the ethical realm requires that one develop a sense of the ending. To envision possible endings is the obligatory prelude to choosing one.

A narrative approach to bioethics focuses on the patients themselves: these are the moral agents who enact choices. Theirs are the lives ruptured by the *peripeteia*, or the transformative event, that the cases highlight. The descriptions, analyses, and interpretations of their journeys through the moral realms of illness become our tradition, our storied past, the collectively held touchstones that enable us to know what to do next. Known to us in rich, earthy, singular complexity, these stories of individual patients form our professional canon, both in ethics and in clinical medicine.

We begin this collection of essays with the transforming realization that the patients are the true ethicists. We professionals accompany them, for sure, with diagnostic help, therapeutic moves, and ethical recommendations. Yet, those who shoulder the duties to act ethically and live with the consequences of their actions are the patients and not their ethicists. Perhaps another result of narrative ethics' emergence will be the realization that, for patients and their families, the ethics under question are not located primarily in the technical questions of providing or withholding health care, allocating scarce resources, or preserving autonomy in the face of death. Those are ethicists' ethical considerations. In large part, the ethics in question are the ethics of ordinary life: how to fulfill life goals, to honor obligations, and to make sense of events in ways that make it possible to go on. These ethical issues have not only to do with *bioethics*; they are also the *ethics of life*.

We open the book with a section that locates the work of bioethicists within a universal search for authentic human communion through language and an effort to create meaning in our lives. Part 2 focuses on the conceptual frameworks from literary studies that ethicists and caregivers use in their work with patients. Each of the authors in this section has both formal training in literary studies and considerable and varied experience in the work of medical ethics. Their essays reveal the fruitful connections between the basic elements of literary analysis and the work they do with ethics cases. Part 3 presents the practice of narrative ethics in its clinical particularities. Five practitioners write about real patients, having gained permission where necessary to publish these essays. In each, the conceptual frameworks of the preceding sections are put to work with an honesty and rigor that have inspired the editors' grateful awe during the writing of this book. Each author reveals the sometimes unexpected utility and transformative power he or she found in bringing narrative methods to bear in clinical work with patients. Part 4 examines explicitly some of the consequences of the practice of narrative ethics for our institutions, our training programs, and our notion of what, indeed, qualifies as ethics. The writers in Part 5 then step forward to *do* the work of bioethics now informed by narrative considerations, letting us see what kinds of questions can be asked and what kind of work can be done with these new methods.

Hourglass in shape, the book starts with generalizations, then narrows—with the help of specific conceptual frameworks from literary studies—to examine very closely one particular story at a time, and then broadens, benefitting from what has been learned from each story to reach a newly achievable plane of realizations about the implications of narrative methods for the work of ethics in medicine. Common themes emerge from the collection of essays that reflect wider and wider circles of signification: the relationship between emotion and reason in moral deliberation, the ethical importance of witnessing the suffering of others, the fundamentally relational nature of understanding between human beings, the possibility of reconciling the inevitable gaps between subjectivity and objectivity, the liminal aspects of illness, and the possibilities for personal transformation open to patients, ethicists, and caregivers. Indeed, the boundaries that generally separate our clinical domains from ethical domains are revealed to be permeable: the same sets of concerns and sources of illumination come to hand whether a doctor treats a patient or an ethicist deliberates about a consultation. The practice of narrative ethics may provide an unforeseen dividend in the new clarity it may give regarding the relations between clinical practice and bioethical practice. We recognize that we are all trying, clinically or ethically, to heal.

Finally, we recognize that individual sick persons and their families are the occasions for vision and insight for us all. As we guide our patients through the ethical rapids and as we come to understand what the moral life requires, we can grow in our own wisdom and usefulness by undergoing formative, authentic encounters with those we hope we serve. Each of us develops his or her own casuistic canon of exemplars of the moral life, regarding that which we witness not necessarily as puzzles to solve but mysteries to behold. Reciprocal and reflective, the practice of narrative ethics demands vision and courage, all the while replenishing one's store of vision and courage. We hope that the communal efforts of this book will embolden us all toward as yet unimaginable bravery, as yet unseen beneficence in the service of patients and their families.

NOTE

1. See Murray Kreiswirth, "Trusting the Tale: The Narrativist Turn in the Human Sciences," *New Literary History* 23 (1992): 629–57; Murray Kreiswirth, "Merely Telling Stories? Narrative and Knowledge in the Human Sciences," *Poetics Today* 21, no. 2 (2000): 293–318; and Donald E. Polkinghorne, *Narrative Knowing and the Human Sciences* (Albany: State University of New York Press, 1988) for discussions of the narrativist turn in several humanities and social science disciplines. See Wallace Martin, *Recent Theories of Narrative* (Ithaca: Cornell University Press, 1986) for a précis of contemporary literary narratology.

PART I

NARRATIVE KNOWLEDGE

CHAPTER 1

NARRATIVES OF HUMAN PLIGHT:
A CONVERSATION WITH JEROME BRUNER
JEROME BRUNER

P rofessor Jerome Bruner met with *Stories Matter* editor (RC) in March 2001 for a conversation about the role of narrative knowledge and practice in medicine and ethics. Professor Bruner introduced the concepts of narrative knowledge to us all in his seminal studies *Actual Minds, Possible Worlds* and *Acts of Meaning.*[1] His formulations of the structure and function of narratives have revolutionized cognitive psychology and the teaching of law, among many other fields. His new book *Making Stories: Law, Literature, Life* discovers how our deepest notions of the self are organized and enacted narratively.[2] Here he speaks about the unity and the meaning of ordinary living achievable through narrative acts, and he suggests narrative means by which bioethicists can improve their practice.

RC: Medicine and bioethics have followed psychology and law and so many other fields in coming around to respecting the power of narrative and trying to understand how it works in our lives. We have begun to examine how narrative competence might help to make our work with sick and dying people more humanistic and more ethically discerning. Help us understand what narrative knowledge is and why we need to know about it.

JB: However specialized the culture, the fact remains that, whatever the specialized job you do, whether it's riveting bolts or taking care of people on death row, there's some kind of underlying thing that gives a kind of unity and sympathy and possibility for the human condition continuing. You're constantly in the process of making narratives. You meet some guy, he said this and did that, and so on. We're always trying to control them by making them sound as if they're something other than narratives. I laugh when people say, "Those are just stories, just narrative, let's get the facts!" We live by stories, and they're what give sense to our lives. We're such biosocial creatures anyway that they may be part of what gives us our biology. They give us a lot of the biology having to do with health. Of course, you have to figure out something about the dosage—you can't give too much! The dehumanizing process first gets expressed as people being rational—I'm not rational about the people I love or hate! I don't have to justify my loyalty to narrative, I just want to let it come into work, not because of the fact that it's self-indulgent on my part, but because human society cannot run without it. And I feel very strongly that rather than talking about stories as old wives' tales, we had better look technically at what on earth they do.

RC: How do we live by stories, and how do stories confer unity?

JB: Telling stories is an astonishing thing. We are a species whose main purpose is to tell each other about the expected and the surprises that upset the expected, and we do that through the stories we tell. In my early studies, to go way back, I was interested in perception and selectivity. We're constantly scanning the world selectively in order to minimize surprise but also to find the kind of thing we're looking for. Now, it was physiologist and Nobelist Lord Adrian who first got me off on this kind of thing. He said, you know, the thing that's so interesting about the reticular system is that it goes "Boom!" when something violates expectancy, and what it does is to clear all the residual and vagrant impulses in the cortex so that by the time the surprising message gets there, it can be heard.

I suppose stories are analogous to the reticular system. We start out with some sort of canonical expectancies of what the world is like, how things are going to be, and then all of a sudden things happen differently; you have what Aristotle referred to as the *peripeteia*. Something knocks expectancy galley west, off course; all of a sudden, you get cancer, your wife leaves you, or your accountant calls to say that the market dropped like mad during the night and you have no money left. There's the *peripeteia*, and then you try to cope with the *peripeteia* and to restore a new legitimacy and expectancy in life. Now what's striking about the new kind of legitimacy on the medical side is that usually, as narrowly defined, the upset of expectancy is, "I've got news for you, you're on the brink of death." The ordinary canonicity is that you'll go on living forever, and now somebody tells you it's finite and you're going to be dead.

RC: And what helps people restore legitimacy after these upsets?

JB: We deal with these upsets—we begin to form a style. We talk about someone—say, Bill; he never panics, he always thinks about how this might have been, what he would do—and we say that's how he is himself. So the great thing is that when people come to this stage of being patients, when they come to the likes of you at the hospital and you have to tell them some hard news that you don't know if they'll make it or not, the person wants to deal with it in some way that has some stylistic integrity about it. That is to say, that's true to them, that's true to the people they love, what the people expect of them. I was thinking of something from Rainer Maria Rilke, "A Death of Your Own." Do you know that piece? It's fantastic, it's about this old man who's having a death of his own. It's real Rilke: it destroys your sleep for three nights afterward. It has to do with death, but it has to do with other things, such as the important turning points in your life. You want somehow to relate your death to what you think of as your itinerary, that your death is going to be like your life in some way. Your death is going to be like your life, the two are going to be of a piece.

RC: Some of us in bioethics have begun to conceptualize our narrative work as trying to do exactly that—helping people to answer the question "In the face of this life, what constitutes a good death?" Can relative strangers help a person to do that?

JB. Well, it's a funny thing. I'll tell you one experience that didn't have to do with death but with blindness for me. I was born blind because of cataracts. Fortunately, they were not opaque, so the light got to my retina. My cataracts were removed by a brilliant surgeon. So I got that done, and well. I've even won a few minor squash championships in my time. I went to the Eye Institute at the Columbia-Presbyterian Medical Center in 1950, because I noticed that a secondary membrane was growing into the place where the lens had been taken out. And I went to a renowned doctor named Doctor Drake, who had a big reputation. I went to him. He said, "It's going to be a bit tricky because we have to go far back on your eyeball." My postoperative eyes were covered up for two days. I couldn't tell whether I could see or not. But at the Eye Institute I had a nurse who sensed my anxiety about "Am I blind or am I not blind?" She came in and said to me, "Hi there, blindfold! How are you doing?" I loved that; it was a recognition that I feared I might be blind and not just blindfolded. Her sharing mattered. This was just an ordinary thirty-five-year-old Irish-American nurse. I recall saying to myself, "If she can do it this way on the fly, what's the matter with the rest of us? Can't the rest of us do it too?"

RC: What is the "it" that she did for you?

JB: She *recognized* my human plight and shared it with me. There are plights having to do with death, having to do with love, having to do with power, with wanting to help someone you can't help. Until you get into one of those plights you don't know what torture is. My nurse recognized the fact that I was not just a "patient," I was somebody with plights, a human being. Plights are everywhere, but the important thing is to pick your plight, be true to coping with it. And not just this particular plight, but you go back again over the class of plights that you have lived with and how you make what you're doing now somehow consistent with a style. There's that wonderful Henry James story about that narrator with his plight of the beast in the jungle, his impenetrable blindness, and then the woman who is in a sense complicit in looking at the thing like that.

RC: May Bartram recognizes Marcher's plight, all right, but it isn't a plight you'd want to be left in, and she isn't able to penetrate his blockhead to let *him* recognize it. Aren't there plights, like Marcher's, that you don't want to be true to but rather free from?

JB: Yes, and the freedom usually *comes from* someone else's recognition. I've had some personal experience with kids, for example, who've been in one of those car crashes that shouldn't happen to anybody, and who have survived only because they've got soft bones and youth. Let me tell you that story—right from the start. It starts a few years before I began working with these kids. I was out skiing in Aspen over a Christmas holiday, going easily down the hill. The top crust broke, and I went through, and my knee broke. They finally operated, and I had to do a lot of exercises to recover. Rita, you won't believe this. When you went to do your exercises, they put you into a curtained cell, a nice little cell with linen curtains. You did your exercises alone. It was pretty grim and hard to do. And it was like that for long months of treatment.

Now, let me go back to the kids. Soon after this accident, about two or three months after the operation and the exercises, I sailed my sailboat across the Atlantic. One's pretty immobilized on a sailboat. When I got to the other side (I was on my way to Oxford), I discovered I couldn't move my leg—it was all bound up at the knee. I went to the orthopedics department at the university and they said, "Come up and take a remedial class with us." Classes? Hmm. What did I discover? They had a whole little gang together, some of these injured kids included. So I would get through my exercises right out there in the open, on the floor of the gym, and then I'd watch the kids. And the nurses would come up to a kid and say, "You couldn't have done that a week ago. That's fantastic!" And soon I got to talking with and working with the kids, mostly by telling stories about their progress and how they'd be next week.

So I got to thinking. You set up a local culture, and people cheerfully do handsprings to fit into it. Local cultures are compelling! To me, a culture trades in canonical narrative. Which is, in that case among those kids, we all had a lousy piece of luck. You banged your head, I knocked off my arm. We can manage. Cheryl Mattingly at occupational medicine or occupational science at the University of Southern California recognizes that physical injury is a thing that's best described by narrative because it comes down to a *peripeteia* and how one copes with it narratively and really. They have some kids, for example, who do bear-chasing exercises, some working against the clock, and some imaginatively rowing across an imaginary channel.

RC: And so your plight was joined to the plights of these kids?

JB: I got through my exercises so fast it would take your breath away. I started dreaming up things I could do to help them with their stuff. Especially games we could play, games *they* liked and could identify with. They loved it; so did I.

RC: Well, isn't that an enactment of the kind of interpersonal commitment you write about in *Making Stories*?

JB: There is a puzzle in all of this. The main thing that made, and makes, *human* culture possible is that you feel a commitment to it and, at the same time, maintain a certain autonomy from it. Commitment works because we're able to sense each other's feelings and beliefs—we are intersubjective to a degree: not only that you do certain things but I know your intentions, and you know mine. It is in this deep sense that no man is an island. And your very self depends on this intersubjectivity.

In *Making Stories*, I reviewed the literature on how people characterize the self. What I found is that selfhood rests upon a good story, a plot with Self as the agent that heads somewhere and gives continuity. These self-creating narratives are often modeled on classics or prototypical cultural forms. So we manage to maintain a certain autonomy while at the same time adhering to cultural forms. It is a little miracle.

The *real* thing is that in a culture, life is made possible by friends and close others, and not just by abstract forces. It's the small communities we join or form and the commitments we make to them that shape us. At the start of adolescence, for example, just breaking into adulthood, my pals and I formed the Demon Crew. We souped up outboard engines, stuck them on the back of cockle-shell hulls, and raced them. We even entered the Around Manhattan Race, and, incredibly, our boat won it in Class C. And there was even a picture of Lenny, one of our gang, who had actually driven the boat, in a Mobil Oil ad in a yachting magazine the next winter! Funny how that sort of thing provides a template for subsequent stories. They have enormous metaphoric reach in life.

RC: It's the plots about ourselves and the metaphors we use in telling them that let us see where we are going, or even choose where we are going.

JB: That's what I mean about finding a way.

RC: If the self is a series of stories . . .

JB: certainly a library of stories . . .

RC: . . . c an we learn to recognize the stories of others?

JB: If we hadn't been able to, we never would have made it as a species.

RC: And how do we learn to tell and listen to stories?

JB: In some way, we all get to it naturally. I'm still leaving open the question of *where* we get this kind of sophistication by the time we're three or four or even much younger. Even before children are able to understand or tell stories in language, they enact them and they love enactments staged by others. Maybe this narrativity comes from language itself, I don't know, it doesn't matter.

More interesting is where do people get knowledge of *plights*? I wish I knew the answer to that. I struggle with making my law students recognize that this isn't just a *case*, this is a client in *trouble*. And trouble is a narrative idea. You have to have a story for there to be trouble, Aristotle's *peripetia*, and that requires a notion of normality or canonicity, and so on.

The fact of the matter is that if you look at how people actually live their lives, they do a lot of things that prevent their seeing the narrative structures that characterize their lives. Mostly, they don't look, don't pause to look. Not even when they are doctors and are supposed to be concerned with the life-and-death stories of their patients.

RC: As plights go, that's the rather most extreme one.

JB: To put it mildly, yes.

RC: Even if the problem is not serious, it stands for what ultimately will be. That's why my medical colleagues are so determined to get it right. Some of them would be very nervous to hear you talk about stories of plight, because they, like your law students, believe that there's only one way to get it right. How can we help them understand that my singular recognition of your plight counts?

JB: Even if it's wrong. If I said something crazy and wrong to you, like, "The reason you're involved in this work is your old man is a doctor and you're caught up in a generational guilt trip," you would say, "No, no, no." But at least I'm on the wavelength of getting it. That's important.

RC: So, do we make a series of efforts and get it righter?

JB: It's a funny way you doctors think that you have to get it righter. Some of you get your satisfaction out of being right about how you thought the lab tests would come out. But that's not good enough. After all, you play the very, very important role of being a kind of cherished outsider. Not that you're going to detechnicalize sickness or health care, but you've got to rehumanize it as well—relate it to life. Who on earth wants to practice like a robot? Or turn their patients into robots?

RC: No, it's horribly wearing and demeaning and it doesn't work.

JB: Yet, sometimes it works in odd forms. Byron Goode, the anthropologist, talks about something that works, though in an odd way. It is the subjunctivization of illness, something that physicians do for their patients that can give them considerable comfort by putting them in a twilight zone. For example, when you're not quite sure that someone has an illness, you talk about it using language in the subjunctive—might be, could be, et cetera.

I came on this same idea in an old study of mine in which I did an analysis of James Joyce's stories in *Dubliners*, showing his use of subjunctivization in comparison with a brilliantly written thing by an anthropologist describing the ritual activity of *penitentes* in New Mexico. Beautiful pieces of writing, both of them. Joyce is full of subjunctivization. His is a world of possibilities. That's what doctors sometimes do for their patients too. Byron, in his studies in Turkey, found out the extent to which, when it is not quite clear whether the person is an epileptic, for example, folk doctors deal with it by telling about it subjunctively, that they might have this or might have that, which has fantastic comforting effects. Nobody's cured, but life is made somewhat more possible.

RC: By sidestepping the need for finality. Sort of letting everyone slowly absorb it, if it were to come to pass. Elliot Mishler taught us in his examination of conversations between doctors and patients that what we have a chance to do—and we ordinarily fail at it as doctors—is to absorb the meaning of what patients try to tell us. Doctors can do this if they choose to, and nurses, like your nurse at the Eye Institute, and ethicists as they do clinical consultations.

JB: So you absorb what patients say and then you try to develop it. There's the big overall picture, but the fact of the matter is, there are pictures along the way over and over again. You want to be good at it, for patients or students or friends. It's not only our human responsibility as teachers and doctors and lawyers, it's somehow advantageous. Everywhere you look, you run into the recognition of the fact that a human plight is never an island unto itself. So, what should you do? You connect.

NOTES

1. Jerome Bruner, *Actual Minds, Possible Worlds* (Cambridge, MA: Harvard University Press, 1986); Jerome Bruner, *Acts of Meaning* (Cambridge, MA: Harvard University Press, 1990).
2. Jerome Bruner, *Making Stories: Law, Literature, Life* (New York: Farrar, Straus, and Giroux, 2002).

CHAPTER 2

THE ETHICS OF MEDICINE, AS REVEALED IN LITERATURE
WAYNE BOOTH

T he drama *Wit*, by Margaret Edson, mostly located in a hospital ward, has become one of the most celebrated plays of this decade. The heroine, a middle-aged woman dying of ovarian cancer, reports to the audience both how she is feeling, as she endures each miserable step of her decline and treatment, and how her miseries relate to her professional life as a teacher of literature. She discovers only slowly that the treatment she has been receiving from top doctors is part of the drug research experiment they are aggressively pursuing. The play provides mounting evidence that the doctors care far more about their research results than about her pain and death; it is possible that they have even violated the standard rules about patient consent. As the heroine, Vivian, dies, she leaves her bed, takes off her garments, and appears before us beautifully nude. She has escaped, by dying, from the inhumane treatment of those doctors and various assistants. Only one nurse has exercised genuine "kindness," teaching the teacher that she should have shown more kindness to her own literature students.

We are thus left with a powerful but complex response: grief at Vivian's suffering, relief over her escape, and fury at the cruel behavior of the doctors, who have in scores of ways revealed that they are more interested in pursuing research results than in what she feels or whether she survives.

The play is not just about the ethical issues of medical treatment. It is aggressively "literary"; Vivian constantly celebrates the beauty of John Donne's *Holy Sonnets*,[1] remembering her skillful—and excessively bossy—teaching of students to understand how Donne probes the meaning of death. But though the play never abandons her interest in literature, and in how Donne's work faces the problems of death, its plot depends on our taking an aggressive ethical stance that relates only obliquely to the study of literature. The power of the ending requires us to share, without question, the author's implied judgment that humane, honest, compassionate treatment of patients is ethically far more important than the pursuit of research results. Thus it can be said to impose on us—some serious researchers might say "dogmatically" or "unfairly"—a decisive ethical conclusion about issues that have plagued philosophers forever: When "truth" and "goodness" clash, which should win? Is it immoral to use a patient's life in the pursuit of truth? Though almost everyone would agree that her doctors have behaved immorally if they did not obtain her consent to be an experiment subject, are they genuinely to blame for "using" her to get results that may be a blessing to many future patients?[2]

Once we begin to think seriously about such questions, implicitly raised in many modern literary works, the issues raised can feel overwhelming. In this essay I can touch only briefly on three of them.

Most obvious is a question that has been faced by philosophers and literary critics for millennia: Is any moral judgment defensible as something more than personal preference? Are there moral or ethical judgments that can be considered rational or demonstrable? Though the moral stance of *Wit* is controversial, can the controversy be thought of as serious pursuit of genuine ethical knowledge? Is there any such thing as genuine ethical knowledge? Second, is it legitimate for any critical reader or spectator to intrude his or her moral views upon the judgment of the work's "literary" or "aesthetic" quality? If I decide (as I personally do not) that *Wit*'s ethical stance is wrong, should that decision reduce my judgment that the play is really wonderful, as a work of "art"? On the other hand, if I share the attack on the doctors, is it right to allow that sharing to increase my admiration for the play, as a work of *art*? No spectator who embraces the play escapes that sharing. But is that increased admiration ethically defensible? Third, is it reasonable to claim that "literature," with all its ambiguities, can teach us—whether patients or medical practitioners—essential ethical truths about the world of health, disease, medicine, and right and wrong ways of facing pain and death? (By "literature" I don't mean merely fictional works. I include autobiographies, memoirs, even journalistic accounts, if they have "literary" elements: anecdote, metaphor, stylistic heightening of emotion.)

Underlying my probing of these three points will be the claim that the pursuers of medical ethics have paid far too little attention to the "fact" that some novelists, poets, and dramatists have probed the issues more deeply than most overt "thinkers" have managed to do.[3]

One: How do we face the claim, still offered by many, that *all* ethical and moral judgments are at best subjective, mere statements of preference? For the utter relativists, the moral skeptics, Margaret Edson's "argument," in *Wit*, that it is immoral to deceive and wound a patient in the service of research results—genuine truth—is simply her personal bias. They might even go so far as to suggest that she takes the stance because, since a majority of playgoers will not be doctors, she can count on their sharing her undemonstrable bias, thus increasing the play's success.

The extreme form of this position says that it is never right for you and me to impose our moral judgments on others, since such judgments have no cognitive basis. Judgments about right and wrong are never "factual," in the scientific sense of empirically demonstrable. So what right have I to impose on others my deep conviction that to do or say this or that is just plain wrong, or vicious, or sinful, or unforgivable?

We defenders of moral judgment point out in reply that such skepticism always sneaks in a moral judgment of its own: it is morally *wrong* to impose any moral judgment—except this one. "You are absolutely morally unjustified in your claim that some moral judgments are absolutely justified."

The hard fact is that all of us, even the most extreme overt relativists, practice that kind of imposition. Ever since "Adam and Eve" partook of the fruit, in Africa, millions of years ago, rising above their animal kin and discovering the difference between good and evil, every one of us has known—at least when not exhibiting sheer madness—that *some* actions committed by *some* of our brothers and sisters *ought* to be forbidden, prevented, or punished, or at least proved to be wrong. Ask any skeptic you know whether it would be right to pass a law forbidding the expression, in print or conversation, of his or her skeptical views. The answer might cautiously avoid terms like "moral" or "ethical," but it would reveal that the skeptic is committed to at least one unqualified—and scientifically unprovable—"ought."

This paradox in the extreme skeptical position does not, however, make the problem go away. Ask your skeptical friends whether Timothy McVeigh was morally justified in bombing the federal building in Oklahoma City, and you'll receive a unanimous "no," even if they go on to say that their judgment is merely culturally determined (I'm assuming that readers of this book do not include many of those who, out of deep "moral" opposition to the U.S. government, think McVeigh behaved morally). But if we ask readers of this book whether we as a nation were right in killing McVeigh, we will land in deep controversy—the kind of irresolvable debate that seems to provide evidence supporting the moral skeptics. Neither side can *prove*, factually or scientifically, that the other side is wrong. The best they can do is show statistics about what the death penalty does or does not do in changing behavior.

The skeptics who claim that, because of these ambiguities, ethical judgments can never be called knowledge will always win if we grant that the test of knowledge is demonstrability in the "scientific" sense: no conviction is demonstrable unless it can pass the test of "falsifiability." Many have joined Karl Popper in arguing that we do not really *know* any proposition, unless we know the logical steps that might disprove it if it were untrue. If we do not know that those steps do not in fact falsify it, our proposition is simply personal opinion, in fact guesswork.[4] Only if you know what steps would be required to disprove an assertion, and if your commitment to doubting leaves the assertion standing, can you claim to have knowledge.

The test is a powerful one in dealing with certain problems. I often use it myself in trying to test my own guesses about how literary works are put together: devise more than one hypothesis, and then decide which one is falsifiable.[5] But stated as a universal dogma, it is highly questionable, as Popper himself sometimes seemed to acknowledge. How, we may ask, does one *know* that the method of testing is *in itself* universally valid? Can the criterion itself be put in falsifiable terms according to its own dictum? Obviously not. It is a value judgment on human intellectual operations, put in the form of a factual claim. As a value judgment it is not, according to the criterion itself, falsifiable.

The falsifiability test is self-evidently crippling when applied to our practical lives. If we know only what survives after we have done our best to doubt everything, we are driven to conclude that most defenses of our actions and judgments have no cognitive base whatever, since we must almost always act on propositions that have not been proved in this sense. "How can you argue," a colleague asks me, "that we have an *ethical* command to pursue ethical questions rationally, when you know that none of our ethical judgments can meet the criterion of falsifiability? My moral choices are not really rational because I really cannot *know* anything about them."

He is right, *if* to "know" must mean to be certain, to have scientific proof, to have propositions that have been tested by the criterion of falsifiability. But this is not in fact the choice that we face.

Being reasonable in moral matters is more like a process of systematic assent than systematic doubt. If my wife says, "I have a sudden terrible pain. Call a doctor quick!" I must and will act at once. Only if I have specific reasons to doubt her claim—if I know, for example, that she is a notorious and sadistic practical joker or liar—do I have warrant to intrude doubt into the process of assent. I do not and should not pause for skeptical probings about the moral rule: "when a friend or mate or any human being is in pain, and you have some chance of doing something about it, you have an absolute command to do what you can."[6] I certainly should not take time to rephrase my hypothesis, "she is suffering," into some falsifiable form, probing her body to see if I can really hurt her.

One could of course go on filling whole books with philosophers' efforts to show why some moral judgments, though of course not all, can be counted as knowledge.[7] Unless we can believe that, we will find no moral judgments about literature—or about medical behavior in and out of literature—that can be called any more than personal preference.

In short, in any ethical enterprise, we must share the unfalsifiable conviction that some actions are right and some wrong.

Two: Should we allow our moral judgments to intrude on our judgments of literary quality? Here we encounter even more skepticism. What right have we to impose upon a novel or play our capricious, undemonstrable private judgments of what distinguishes good and bad behavior? Critical discussions through recent decades have been loaded with controversy about whether this or that negative moral judgment can rightly be imposed on a work that is in other respects—in its "artistic"quality—admirable. Is it right to give some negative marks to Shakespeare's *The Merchant of Venice* because it is strongly anti-Semitic?[8] Was it both stupid and unfair of me, as one historian colleague claimed, to raise some "feminist" objections to Rabelais's *Gargantua and Pantagruel*?[9] Am I right to praise *Wit* in part because of its ethical stance about one kind of medical research?

Though it may seem a bit remote from my basic subject here, it may prove useful to consider the question of whether our judgments about right and wrong sexual practice should be allowed to influence our aesthetic judgments. A scientific study I have not conducted reveals that 79 % of all modern novels include at least one sexual act that 55.5 % of readers consider immoral. Only 25.4 % of those novels reveal clear moral judgments by the narrator or implied author. All the others leave all judgment up to the reader.

All jesting aside, I find it revealing that so few modern novels—unlike those of earlier centuries—reveal explicit judgment about whether any of the innumerable sex acts are morally indefensible. When Henry James, in *The Ambassadors*, shows his hero Lambert Strether discovering that the relationship between Chad Newsome and Mme. de Vionnet, which he had considered mere friendship, is actually illicit adultery, the reader has never a doubt but that the author himself joins Strether in condemning the adultery.[10] But when the heroes of most novels these days roam about the sexual landscape indiscriminately, there is seldom any strong hint about whether the author draws any lines between what's admirable, what's acceptable, and what's contemptible. The chief exceptions are novels, mostly by women, in which women or children are sexually abused; almost all authors and readers agree that when an adult rapes a child, a genuinely evil act has occurred. Is that judgment demonstrable, by the standards employed by some skeptics? Obviously not.

Consider the less dramatic question of whether a professor's or doctor's sexual pursuit of a student or patient is ever defensible. In three novels I've recently read—and there are probably scores more—the hero/professor has sex with a girl student. In Robert Hellenga's *The Fall of a Sparrow*,[11] the protagonist, a professor of English, has sex with a beautiful "foreign" student, is discovered, and is kicked out by his college. All of the moral judgments by the implied author, many made explicit by the narrator, are against the college administrators for their blind moralism. There is not a word about the ethical conflict between lust and abuse of academic power. And there is no hint that the protagonist thinks he has committed an act genuinely subject to ethical objection.

In J. M. Coetzee's *Disgrace*, we find a somewhat more honest confrontation. A South African professor of English is caught imposing sex upon a beautiful student enrolled in his "Romantic Literature" course. When he first proposes that she "spend the night" with him, she asks "Why?" and he answers, "Because you ought to."

> "Why ought I to?"
> "Why? Because a woman's beauty does not belong to her alone. It is part of the bounty she brings into the world. She has a duty to share it...."
> "And what if I already share it?"...
> "Then you should share it more widely."[12]

She resists this first advance and leaves him. The author then intrudes a moral judgment against his protagonist: "That is where he ought to end it." But the "hero" does not. He goes on pursuing her. And shortly later, he forces sex on her. "She does not resist. All she does is avert herself; avert her lips, avert her eyes."

And then come the ambiguous moral judgments (it's not entirely clear whether the author intends to share them with the hero): "Not rape, not quite that, but undesired nevertheless, undesired to the core. As though she had decided to go slack, die within herself for the duration...." When she then sends him away, "He obeys, but then, when he reaches his car, is overtaken with such dejection, such dullness, that he sits slumped at the wheel unable to move.

"A mistake, a huge mistake. At this moment, he has no doubt, she, Melanie, is trying to cleanse herself of it, of him" (p. 25).

After more sexual encounters, the scandal of it hits the campus, and he is, like the hero of Hellenga's novel, kicked out by the administration. The reader is not left, as in Hellenga's hands, with no hint of any moral problem; the implied author obviously shares the hero's regrets about his "mistakes." But there is no clear encounter with the question: Why is it wrong for a professor to succumb to lust with one of his students? And of course there is no hint about whether reader Booth is wrong to admire Coetzee more than Hellenga, *as artist*, because he at least addresses the moral issues.[13]

For a third example, consider Philip Roth's latest book, *The Dying Animal*, now receiving mixed reviews.[14] Even though I knew that it would be full of sexual encounters, I expected no moral judgments about it. Most of Roth's earlier works provide little hint that fulfilling certain kinds of lustful drive can be judged as vicious. In this book, very early on, to my surprise, after the hero-narrator reports how sexually attractive he finds one of his students, he suddenly inserts what sounds like a strong moral judgment, one that could be taken as a critique of Hellenga and even of Coetzee:

> Now, I have one set rule of some fifteen years' standing that I never break. I don't any longer get in touch with them [my female students] on a private basis until they have completed their final exam and received their grade and I am no longer officially in loco parentis. In spite of temptation—or even a clear-cut signal to begin the flirtation and make the approach—I haven't broken this rule since, back in the mid-eighties, the phone number of the sexual harassment hotline was first posted outside my office door. (p. 5)

But then he quickly wipes out what has appeared as a *moral* code and turns it into a "set rule" that is mere self-protection: "I don't get in touch with them any earlier so as not to run afoul of those in the university who, if they could, would seriously impede my enjoyment of life" (p. 5).

And of course he never gets caught and kicked out of his teaching position: he has adopted not a moral code but a self-protective code, with almost no hint, throughout the book, of how his aggressive pursuits of woman after woman has harmed them (he feels harmed himself, when one of them leaves him for another lover, but who cares how much he hurts them?). His infidelities are simply the product of a lust that, by implication, *ought not* to be inhibited except when it might get him into trouble.

Of course no reader can be sure whether Roth intends us to join the narrator's views with his implied author's moral positions. It could be that Roth is mocking his hero for *pretending* to make a moral judgment that is really only an act of self-protection. We'll never know.

I bring in these three non-medical examples to dramatize the question: Do I believe that their different ways of addressing or ignoring moral questions should affect our judgment about the *aesthetic* quality of each novel? Yes, of course. For me, Coetzee rises a bit above the others because he addresses moral issues throughout. But do I think that Hellenga's and Roth's reveling in student sex, without a hint of moral inquiry, *utterly* destroys their aesthetic quality? Of course not; it only diminishes but need not destroy my admiration. It is simply that I learn more about life when an author like Coetzee or Henry James takes me into his way of coping with the ambiguities and tensions that moral judgments lead to. James teaches me more about how to grapple with moral complexities than any formal philosopher I have read.

Three: When we turn from ethical criticism of all kinds of literature back to literature that deals with medical problems, we meet similar issues—issues that are not as widely discussed as are those about sex. How can literature, when dealt with *ethically*, teach us more not just about sexual morality but about how doctors and patients *should* live—more than we learn from the handbooks concerning medical ethics?

Well, as readers here know, there has been a flood of novels and memoirs written—mainly by those who have faced life-threatening disease—addressing ethical problems of medicine. Most of them are written from the patient's point of view, often revealing just how much difference can result from the diverse ethical stances that doctors take as they perform their treatments. And too many of them, from my "moralistic" perspective, follow Hellenga and Roth in failing to address the complex issues that their stories reveal. However, unlike Hellenga and Roth, they work hard to underline this or that moral point, ignoring the ambiguities and complexities.

The possible candidates for the role of "genuine educators about medical ethics and the ethics of dying" are innumerable. Tolstoy's "The Death of Ivan Ilych," Richard Powers's *Gain* or *Wandering Soul*, Pat Barker's *Regeneration*, Saul Bellow's *Ravelstein* (the final section, really a report on Bellow's own illness), Reynolds Price's *A Whole New Life: An Illness and a Healing*, François Mauriac's *Knot of Vipers*, and so on.

For the sake of brevity, consider a brilliant recent novel now receiving rave reviews, David Lodge's *Thinks....*[15] Because the heroine and her would-be lover dispute, often quite profoundly, about the contrast between literary and scientific treatment of human consciousness, the whole book could be considered relevant to this essay. But I must concentrate on only one moment, hoping that my discussion will not spoil the book's plot for those who have not yet read it. Helen, the novelist who has to her own surprise finally fallen in love with Messenger, the dogmatically mechanistic cognitive scientist, suddenly learns that he may have fatal liver cancer. In their long discussions of how to deal with his illness, she is shocked by his request that if the diagnosis turns out to be positive, she must, if she loves him, provide some kind of assisted suicide. He insists that he will not face the miseries of extended painful and pointless treatment of the kind the heroine of *Wit* received.

> "I don't want to put up a brave fight. I don't want to be ill for a year or two and then die, helpless, wasted, incontinent, bald. No thanks....As soon as I'm quite sure...I shall make for the Exit while I'm still able to walk out unassisted. Well, perhaps not entirely unassisted."

He then requests her help, and she is horrified by his request.

> "Messenger, this is horrible. I don't want to listen any more."
> "I thought you wanted to help me."
> "What do you want me to do then?" she says, her voice rising. "Hold a plastic bag over your head? Kick the stool away from under your feet?"

After rising emotion on both sides,

> "I'm not joking, Helen."
> "No, I wish you were," she said. "What about the distress to me?"
> "I know I'm asking a lot. But it would be an act of . . . of love."
> "*Love?*" Helen laughs, a little hysterically.

And after a bit more arguing about the issues, she flatly refuses, concluding with "Messenger, it's *because* I love you" (pp. 282–83).

So here we have two forms of genuine love in genuine ethical conflict about disease and death: "Kill me if you love me"; "I won't kill you, because I love you." The conflict is addressed in a way that only powerful literature can achieve.

In all of the public controversy about assisted suicide, and about the imprisonment of Kervorkian, I've seen very little serious inquiry of the Lodge kind into how we might think and feel, or *learn* to think about feelings and about the ethical issues doctors and patients face when dealing with aging and life-threatening disease. The ethical stances are, apparently for a majority, clearly on Helen's side: "It's morally wrong to commit suicide, under any circumstances." "It's morally vicious, even criminal, to assist in suicide." Apparently a small, if growing, minority falls on the other side: "It's obviously wrong to prolong a miserable painful life when the patient herself prefers death." But the tiniest minority is of those who, like Lodge, feel the importance of grappling with the emotional issues, on both sides.

It remains frustrating, of course, that attending to those who do the serious grappling will never provide us with decisive answers. Though most authors will finally take some kind of firm stand, attending to them will still leave us having to *think* (borrowing Lodge's title), giving serious attention to the arguments and feelings on both "sides" of any ethical dispute.

From all this we can extract no clear moral code, no list of Seven Rules for Effective Medical Use of Literature. But as I conclude without a firm, decisive, clear conclusion, you may finally detect four implicit messages underlying this whole essay.

First, every creative author who portrays serious illness ought to move openly and aggressively into the moral issues faced by both the patient and the doctor, carefully avoiding oversimplified embrace of only one side. Simply to portray one clear "side" in any issue may feel good and may make readers feel good, but it can fail to encourage ethical *thinking*. On the other hand, when a really thoughtful play like *Wit* takes its firm stand, but portrays persuasively the characters on the other "side," it can encourage thinking—especially in those who start on the "wrong" side. Similarly, *Think*... will lead any careful reader to be more skeptical about arguments regarding assisted suicide—at least of the more selfish kinds.

Second, every medical practitioner should attend more closely to the stories patients (or their literary creators) are telling and have told about how it has felt to be treated this way and that way, as the patient has faced possibly fatal illness or the aging that will inevitably prove fatal.

Third, doctors and nurses should think hard about how their behavior *feels* to the patient. Ethical questions are not just about the large issues I have discussed but also about how the character projected by the practitioner affects the quality of the life of the patient.[16] The sympathetic nurse Suzie, in *Wit*, appalled by the doctors' lack of feeling, actually takes Vivian's hand, after one doctor has declared that she's finally "out of it," and rubs it with baby oil. The widespread practice of silence about ethical matters, the simple habit of implying that to bring ethics into a conversation about literature or about medicine rules out serious inquiry and genuine knowledge, must be attacked on all fronts.[17]

The knowledge we can hope for will not be the kind that hard science will embrace (except in those rare cases where *genuine* statistical studies are employed). It will rather be the kind of knowledge that comes when, after time spent seriously *thinking together* and reading important literary portrayal of medical crisis, we arrive at convictions that we know are true, because we can think of no reasons to question them. Instead of the "falsifiability" criterion and the rhetoric of total skepticism ("Only if I can disprove, scientifically, all of the possible doubts I can raise"), we need a rhetoric of assent: "If I feel that I *know* that this standard is real, and if I can find no solid reasons for doubting it, after serious probing of the other side, it is real." I may find reasons to question it, down the line, but until then, I should do my best to win others into my camp, while listening closely to their efforts to win me into theirs.

Fourth and finally, an even more dogmatic assertion: the medical world should pay more attention to works like *Wit* and *Gain* and *Regeneration*. Though they cannot *demonstrate* absolutely that certain medical practices are wrong, they can, if experienced genuinely in their emotional power, force every doctor or nurse to think just a bit harder before embracing this or that form of medical practice.

NOTES

1. In a longer essay I might well use Donne's sonnets as "proof" of the value, in medical thinking, of literary probing.

2. As I write, in July 2001, the most talked about controversy of this kind is about stem cell research on embryos. But the issues are radically different when both research truth and human good are on one side—the value of the research in saving lives—and only a minority see "the good" as entirely on the side of preserving the embryo.

3. I must confess that I have read only a tiny fraction of what is called "medical ethics." But that fraction has revealed hardly anything about how literature might contribute to the inquiry.

4. Karl Popper, *Logik der Forschung*, trans. as *The Logic of Scientific Discovery* (London, 1959; 2nd ed. 1968).

5. I make use here of some statements from my book, *Modern Dogma and the Rhetoric of Assent* (Chicago: University of Chicago Press, 1974), 101–111, on "systematic doubt" and "systematic assent."

6. The philosophical and religious versions of this moral rule could more than fill this article. For me the most penetrating is Kant's categorical imperative, a universal rule that might well be seen as a justification for the Hippocratic oath. It can be summarized as a version of the Golden Rule that avoids the dangers of thinking only of one's preferences. "Do unto others as you would have others do unto you" has been interpreted by some critics as saying: "Get what you can from others, by treating them well." Kant's version is, in effect: "Always try to act in a way that you think all human beings should act. Treat the welfare of every person as an inviolable *end* or purpose of life." How could anyone ever apply the falsifiability test to that one?

7. One of the best brief defenses of the rationality of moral choice is Bernard Williams's *Morality: An Introduction to Ethics* (New York: Harper and Row, 1972). Most of the major philosophers have provided much more extensive "defenses," from Plato and Aristotle on. One of my favorites is Spinoza's *Ethics*. Too many even of these defenses pay too little attention to the "casuistical" problems that arise when "cases" produce a clash between unquestionable, universally valid values. All defenders of moral values must finally rely on a pluralistic (not utterly relativistic) embrace of diverse forms of defense. For my most recent effort in this direction, see "Relativism, Pluralism, and Skepticism from a Philosophical Perspective," in *International Encyclopedia of the Social and Behavioral Sciences* (Oxford: Elsevier Science, 2001).

8. I grapple with this and other examples in "Why Banning Ethical Criticism Is a Serious Mistake," *Philosophy and Literature* 22 (October 1998): 366–93. I can assume that most readers here strongly oppose anti-Semitism. And most would agree that the

basic plot of *The Merchant of Venice* is anti-Semitic, even though Shakespeare includes some genuinely humane moments. But I wonder how many readers would agree that it is legitimate to reduce one's *aesthetic* admiration for the play because Shakespeare allows himself to fall into a cultural judgment almost universal in his time.

9. Of course some feminists have argued that I didn't go far enough; I unconsciously revealed male chauvinism even as I claimed to do feminist criticism. I resist intruding the data here.

10. For an excellent probing of the moral ambiguities and judgments in James's novels, see Robert Pippin, *Henry James and Modern Moral Life* (Cambridge: Cambridge University Press, 2000).

11. Robert Hellenga, *The Fall of a Sparrow* (New York: Scribner, 1998).

12. J. M. Coetzee, *Disgrace* (New York: Viking Press, 1999), 16. Subsequent page references to this work appear in parentheses in the text.

13. A much superior novel in many respects is his *The Sixteen Pleasures* (New York: Soho Press, 1994).

14. Philip Roth, *The Dying Animal* (New York: Scribner, 2001). Page references to this work appear in parentheses in the text.

15. David Lodge, *Thinks…* (New York: Viking, 2001). Page numbers appear in parentheses in the text.

16. See the essay "Reconsidering Action: Day-to-Day Ethics in the Work of Medicine," by John Lantos, chapter 16 in this volume.

17. There you observe *my* moral dogma.

CHAPTER 3

LIKE AN OPEN BOOK: RELIABILITY, INTERSUBJECTIVITY, AND TEXTUALITY IN BIOETHICS
LAURIE ZOLOTH AND RITA CHARON

But is not the secret of the face the other side of the different way of thinking—
one more ambitious, and presenting a different configuration than that of
knowledge/thinking?

　　　　　　　　　　　　　—Emmanuel Levinas, "The Meaning of Meaning"

INTRODUCTION

A friend of mine, a young anthropologist, once told me, Zoloth, about her work. She had done field research on a tribe who had left the wars of Central America, and, for several generations, had lived in a remote jungle in the Northeastern corner of South America. I was struck by her account that the tribe had no word and no concept for narrative fiction. Stories were either "true" or they were "a lie." After a few years of watching the tribe and answering questions about her American life for them, she brought a VCR and videotapes of popular films to the village as a little present. The villagers watched politely, and then inquired about the subsequent health of the people in the story; perhaps they were her friends? And when she told them that the whole thing, the drama, the emotions, the courageous actions, the love, had all been, well, *made up* to tell a story, they were appalled. They tried to teach their children not to lie—what was this? It was not that they lacked narrative forms: they were a complex sort of Christian and had what we would call mythic origin stories—how the rocks and rivers had come to be, who the ancestors were, and the story of the Resurrection in a slightly altered South American version. But these narratives were considered true, of course—the gospel truth.

What they did not have, or hold as valuable, were Shakespeare, Dickens, and Faulkner, or oral fictions of pretend persons. The company of the fictive, by which we in Western culture come to know and to assess the morality and courage of our own stories, collectively and personally, was entirely absent. But in all other ways, she told me, life was the same. Food was gathered and cooked, celebration was made, love, children, death, choice, all the same, only without the lies we love to whisper to one another, or to read aloud. Or to live by.

TRUTH CLAIMS AND TRUE LIES

We feel baffled by the paradox of this ethnographic report because we so love our stories, and we claim that our literary accounts have the power to tell us the truth. This is the premise of teaching literature, of course, and the premise of narrative ethics as a method to reveal the veracity under the illusion of the mutable case stories in medicine. One of the largest claims made by such a method is that narrative texts and methods can inform the decisions faced in the world of bioethical dilemmas. We argue in our teaching that the fictional story (not really real) can help us confront the terrible starkness of the irrefutably real clinical impasse, because narrative, and the way we understand it, allows us to see moral claims in action, allows us alliances, cases, and language for the confrontation. It is a claim that needs defending—not only to the tribe of Mayans, but to the discourse of medical ethics in which narrative ethics seeks to make such a claim. The claim is not unfamiliar: it is central to the research of several fields. Bioethicists are learning, as the field matures, how to garner and distinguish the news of the world from the variant sources of context, argument, linguistic complexities, and daily praxis. Hence, we will argue in this chapter for an emergent theory of narrative bioethics based on two voices and two disciplines—literary theory (Charon) and textual reasoning in philosophy (Zoloth).

THE RESPONSIBILITY OF THE CASE STORY

If literary studies have the power to inform decisions in bioethics, it is because the knowledge of the self and others entered through the serious engagement with stories in literature is pivotal in thinking about case stories in ethics. The narrative ethics practiced by some literary scholars, unrelated to bioethics though arising in the same time period and context, can help us to examine this claim. Literature's narrative ethics examines the reciprocal responsibilities incurred by the writer who encodes thoughts and feelings into language and by the reader who rescues from words their secrets.[1] Writer and reader (or teller and listener) develop deep powers and daring intimacies as they meet in text, for the writer, however cannily or uncannily, reveals aspects of the self while the reader, with whatever skill is available, penetrates the text toward that which put it into motion. This literary brand of narrative ethics guides the textual actors toward mutual respect and comprehension while governing the potential for exploitation or expropriation whenever one opens oneself to penetration by another.

Although the *content* of our stories—the deceit in "The Death of Ivan Ilych" or love in the face of death in *The Magic Mountain*—indeed helps bioethicists understand what might be the fitting and moral path of action in a bioethical dilemma, the processes we undergo in reading them may be more contributory. What happens when a reader engages with a text? Some readers deploy what literary critic Denis Donoghue has called *graphi-reading*, a sort of reading that treats the text not as a window to a human presence "behind" the language (and thereby inferring an absence), but as a virtuality, an immediacy, a plenitude. Such reading, championed by the deconstructionists, posits not the author or reader or subjects but the language itself as the hero of the text, enforcing semiotic play and embarrassed by human sentiment. Another kind of reading, *epi-reading*, can be conceptualized as an occasion of authentic meetings between persons. "We read a poem," writes Donoghue in *Ferocious Alphabets*, "not to enlighten ourselves but to verify the axiom of presence: we read to meet the other."[2] Reader and writer are engaged in a process of recognition, reconciliation, and reflexive transformation in the acts of giving and receiving text. Instead of seeing reading and writing as acts of communicating semiotic messages, the epi-reader calls it communion. "Each person describes or tries to make manifest his own experience: the other, listening, cannot share the experience, but he can perceive it, as if at a distance."[3] Using such a reading model to interrogate the work of the ethicist helps to examine—and then to choose among alternatives—the stance of the teller, the position of the listener, and how they might best relate to one another. Even more than with their answers, such models help us with their questions: What relationships do narratives create? How does a story work on those influenced by it? What has changed by virtue of the story being told? How can one ever know what a story means?

Like reading stories in literature and reasoning after the book is closed, reasoning about case stories in bioethics relies on the claim—at least the provisional claim while within the text's presence—that the world of the other is true. What one seeks in moral reflection about the bioethics case is not only a provisional solution to the question "What is a fitting action in this situation?" but also, more elegantly, "What is this world I have entered?" (That the anterior and altogether more savage question "How ought I to live?" is also always mobilized is to say that the insistence of the ethical demand is also a constant.) The conversation one has with another—the patient, the family, the nurse, the intern—rests on the intersubjective pact, that is, the agreement that one is not completely alone in interpreting this construction of reality. One stands oneself as a sign for the other, making room in the reasoning, with risk and utter trust, for the interpretation offered by another. In the clinical world, of course, such pacts are complicated by and implicated in the vulnerability of illness, the power asymmetries in hospitals, and the little time there usually is in which to act. And yet at all times and in all cases, the intersubjective pact requires one's *presence*, that is to say, one's humble participation in the work at hand—it will be what slows, stabilizes, and disrupts the givenness of power as the case is first and quickly told.

Something of this same claim is made by the use of textual analysis and textual reasoning in philosophy, in which the word stands as signification of a world of interlocking, intertextually linked events. The text opens into multiple meanings, each derivative of possible narrative interpretations, which in turn depend on the creation of a shared interpretive community built around the text—hence the claim is that the text is "written" by its interpretation. Noting in this method the traces of one-to-another, the philosopher is led to see the reversibility of the self and the other. Literary studies and philosophic reasoning can propose to understand the case story of the clinic, then, as a reciprocity of case and story and to see in the confrontation of stories the reversibility of self and other. It is only this willingness to submit to such vulnerability and similarity that allows a moral argument to be made.

ESTRANGEMENT AND ENGAGEMENT: THE TURN TOWARD PARTICULARS

Issues of identity, boundaries, and social terrain vex bioethics and its methods. Decades after having been inaugurated as a profession, bioethics continues to ask identity questions. If we are strangers at the bedside, and if we are asked there precisely because we are not practicing clinical medicine, then how is it that we remain outside the discourse yet are engaged social actors responsible for the moral gestures we enact? Having been called into being *because* of our difference from those who do the work of health care and those who have the health care done to them, we now find ourselves reassessing the value of exactly that remoteness that, at the start, was our singular merit.

We think we are meant to represent a point of view, a body of knowledge, a set of principles, an authority to adjudicate differences in opinion or action. And yet, the world of the clinical ethicist, unlike the world of philosophers and legal theorists and literary scholars of the academy, is one of particularities. It is our place to be at the bedside, a lucky verticality that answers a horizontality, a self that is able to leave yet that hears grief, chance, and suffering. While there at the bedside, we feel the tension of our estrangement and the necessity of our engagement while we register the plight of those suffering disease and those suffering with the responsibility for caring for the sick. Our moral arguments are preceded by the moral gesture of this accountability, this essential responsibility we carry because we are free (for now) to leave the room and the hard choices of mortality to return to the world of the outside. It is the tension between our narrative positions—the necessary strangerliness of the watching bioethicist,[4] and the desperation of the particular individual patient whom we see—that reveals much about our theory and intellectual frameworks, and that, without the particulars, would remain hidden, thematized, and safely obscured.

Once we begin to work on a case, the principles and the tenets are perforce transformed by the particulars of *this one* case. In his work on the theory of narrative in bioethics, Tod Chambers reminds us that we perform the moral gesture of bioethics consultation only by way of cases, and cases are stories of the tangible, embodied world, however abbreviated their form and however contrived their genre. The tools we need—and so need to teach—to perform as ethicists not only derive from analytic philosophy, although such capacities as the search for relevant principles and the recognition of normative duties are essential. We also need such tools of literary perceptions as "reportability," "closure," "characters," "chronotype," and "gender."[5] By paying attention to how the story works on us, we see more clearly where we are in the story, and this ultimately shows us something like the way out of the case, the denouement, the door back to the outside world. If seeing the case, like reading works of literature, is a reawakening in us of other stories, then the moral argument of bioethics proceeds only by way of particular, and intertextually verified, stories.

This turn toward the particular instance is destabilizing for a bioethics that considers itself a juridical enterprise. Taking into account the particular, after all, is a habit one is trained to break in science and in the academy. Attention to the particular, one is taught, is a concession to a trompe l'oeil—a weakness, a distraction, a dismissible lapse. Because such attention enmeshes one in the tragic, it is suspect, and it may well be a lie. What one prefers over the anecdotal particular is the replicable veracity, facticity with a large *n*, with consistent numbers, with claims that will always repeat with any patient, with any doctor, because they are true.

Descartes's teachings about the subjective and interpretive nature of objectivity seem salient to this tension between the particular and the universal. "[T]he ability to judge correctly, and to distinguish the true from the false—which is really what is meant by good sense or reason—is the same by innate nature in all men; and...differences of opinion are not due to differences in intelligence, but merely to the fact that we use different approaches and consider different things."[6] Facing the Great Story of Catholic teachings about the natural world, a Bible story that framed all contemporary understanding as surely as popular culture takes hold of our moral imagination today, Descartes entreats us to struggle to doubt everything in the effort to reach to the data itself. Paradoxically, Descartes asserts that subjectivity must derive from one's own direct experience and particular reason while objective truth claims must be personal as well as public, sharable, and justified as reality. How can a truth be both particular and universalizable?

Such a paradox is hard to embrace. Science, made possible by the search for and application of data and the flight from the subjective, is one response. Narrative studies, by privileging the singular and apprehending truth claims interpretively, is another. We two authors insist on both solutions: illness and the ethical response to it contain elements of causality and generalizability side by side with individual and incommensurable meaning. Bearing shared witness to particular, idiosyncratic stories while bringing to bear all that can be known about them are the means by which we move from making single observations to joining a coherent interpretive community that alone allows moral choice.

HEARERS AND TELLERS

The ethicist has to adjudicate not only the claims of the case but the claims on self made by it. To have chosen bioethics is to find oneself undermined, altered, case by case by case, story by story by story, drawn to ever renegotiate one's pact with one's work. The methodological tasks of bioethics demand personal characteristics and behaviors that are not necessarily mobilized in the library or the laboratory—interpersonal attention, acceptance of one's duty toward another, diminishment of one's needs in relation to the needs of the other, and the reversibility of self and other upon which empathy depends. Those who chose bioethics did not necessarily foresee that these aspects of self would be required, and some may find themselves uneasy living a life that requires them. And so one is brought to the question of identity both professionally and personally: How does the encounter with the other alter the construction of the moral community to which one is accountable? How does it alter the nature of the self? What are the implications of the intersubjective pact at the foundation of this work?

The terms of the pact are rigorous. Like in the work of the clinician, the stakes of engagement are high if the work is to be decently done. And like in the work of readers and writers, the outcomes of the venture are mutual. When literary scholar Barbara Herrnstein Smith defined narrative discourse as "*someone telling someone else that something happened*," she signaled the centrality of the intersubjective situation to narrative acts.[7] (Literary scholars and philosophers differ in how they use the word *intersubjective*. Like psychologists or psychoanalysts, literary scholars use the word to refer to the meeting between two authentic selves, not only as they gaze at a third object, but as they develop a relation.) Narrative activity presupposes a relation between at least two singular beings. It is one contribution of narrative theory to bioethics to recognize that moral discernment is a form of narrative activity and that arguments and principles are made within the specificity of particular narratives told by particular tellers to particular listeners. In examining what happens between writers and readers or between tellers and listeners, narrative theory deepens our comprehension of what happens between patients and doctors and between ethicists and those they serve.

Narrative competence endows one with the tools to understand the moral and social consequences of words being transmitted and received. Many recent developments in literary theory—semiotic theory, reader-response criticism, autobiographical theory, and some aspects of poststructuralist thought—assist in the effort to disentangle the meant from the said, the said from the heard, and the heard from the understood. Each of these potential entanglements is, it must be pointed out, both textual and relational. When one subject attempts to convey something to another subject so that it is heard, there is only one avenue for doing so, and that avenue is narrative discourse. (Unlike clinicians, all we in bioethics have to exchange is words.) To effectively convey the simplest thought or feeling—the sky is blue, your shoelaces are untied, I am thirsty, I am afraid—requires the narrative elements of diction, voice, metaphor, syntax, intention, time, form, and desire. Each narrative element can be understood, and each must be understood in order for textual work to proceed. And more: understanding what is conveyed by another relies on the idea that "blueness" and "thirst" have both a social and a moral meaning, and attending to the moral universe in which "thirst" *requires* a response makes the simple exchange a moral exchange.

In the clinical world, stories call for response. As the patient speaks, the ethicist's story of self is ruptured. The ethicist is a moral agent, offering with his or her presence an account that is itself interrogated and interrupted by the discourse of the clinic. As a moral actor in this narrative, the ethicist must answer to the conversation. He or she cannot *tell* or *give recommendations* without this necessity of the imperative interruption. The presence of the ethicist is not the only one required. But the ethical response that is the consultation is imperative: If the encounter fails, if the ethicist is absent, the peril is not only that the course of action cannot be logically evaluated, but also that there is no one who can "read" the text that the patient offers, and centrally, no one who can respond to the deep moral question that is both one of interpretation and one of expectation: Will my thirst be sated? Will my apprehension of beauty, my claim for the blueness of the sky, be supported? Does my claim and my desire—or only my illness—matter in the clinical world?

These acts of transmission and reception join the two subjects—the teller and the listener—in an act of moral interpretation, a word that means, as feminist psychoanalytic critic Julie Kristeva points out, "to be mutually indebted."[8] The ordinal tasks faced in this encounter are thus not only the ones of positivistic science, to measure, to replicate, and to change the direction of the outcome, but also the linguistic efforts to make meaning through mutually interpretive acts. The bioethicist and the moral community become, in the encounter of the ethical dilemma, the expert readers of what are by definition complex, ambiguous, and risky texts. No texts—and these are no exceptions—are told by telling machines, and no texts are read by reading machines. Each of these texts *comes* from somewhere, and each, in order to be understood, goes somewhere. These two "moral locations" are persons, subjects, signs, and stories. And so in the absorptive processes of acts of interpretation, acts that include both the telling and the listening, the two subjects are mutually indebted because each one in the encounter is a sign for the other. As subject, I am queried and interrupted by the presence of another.[9] The demands of the vulnerable patient in the clinical situation of the bioethical dilemma create a heightened level of intensity in this interrogation. The very encounter asks about the worth of the ethicist: Why are you here, who are you, can you help me, what is the warrant for your listening? One's status as a person of authority affiliated with those who own and control the encounter with illness is challenged in this intersubjective relationship. The patient is the vulnerable one, yes, precisely, but she is the one with ontological power in the encounter, for only by her queries can one make the justifying argument of one's being: *who I am* is defined by the encounter with her. Hence the debt of the self toward the patient exists at the most existential level.

THE ENCOUNTER WITH THE OTHER AS RUPTURE: EMMANUEL LEVINAS

To be indebted is to be transformed by the other, and this transformative process renders the speaking self, in the moral geophysical language of location, "higher" than the encountering, listening self. This conceptual and spatial notion in ethics is most fully developed by French Jewish philosopher and Talmudist Emmanuel Levinas. Levinas has become a germinal thinker for bioethicists from both philosophy and literary studies because his work illuminates the transformative and disconcerting implications of listening to the other, hence taking responsibility for the other. Levinas's thought also helps to clarify the particularity of the ethical moment, that is to say, the incommensurability of each relation between subject and other, the impossibility of repeating that which occurs, authentically, between two human beings, and the subtlety of the debt that the philosopher incurs by being in conversation. Like his predecessors Heidegger and Husserl,[10] Levinas considers two aspects of the human problem that lie directly underneath the particularities of the work of the ethicist: our instability about time and our desires about death. It is the ethical encounter with the other that allows us meaning—and in this we understand why the ethics consultation is not only an interpretive act, it is both an ontological and a world-defining activity. It is the "calling into question":

> A calling into question that cannot be interpreted as an event, whether essential or accidental, marking the intrigue of the being of beings. A calling into question in which the question springs forth older than the one about the meaning of the being of beings; a calling into question in which the very problematic nature of the question, perhaps, emerges, not the questionable nature of the question . . . but the question that is counternatural, against the very naturalness of nature: "Is it just to be?"[11]

Levinas understands that the knowledge of another is made possible only by the practicalities of "proximity, of sociality that does not lead back to ontology, and is not based on the experience of being and in which meaning is not defined formally, but by an ethical relation to the other person in the guise of responsibility to him or her" (p. 93). In the encounter with the exposed face of the other (and, we would add, in the heightened starkness of the naked "clinical" body of the other), one comes to confront the secrets of the other that come unannounced through the usual "sign, facial expressions, language and words" (p. 93). One is summoned, claims Levinas, by immediacy, claimed by a responsibility that is "incurred in no previous experience" (p. 94).

THE IMPERATIVES OF TIME AND DEATH

Like any other narrative enterprise, bioethics deals with the fragile temporality of the human condition, the facticity of human time that is both real and a social construct, both invented and inevitable. Frank Kermode's example of a simple narrative is "tick-tock." "*Tick* is a humble genesis, *tock* a feeble apocalypse; and *tick-tock* is in any case not much of a plot."[12] Kermode's least common denominator reflects the temporal truth that, in order for plot to occur—in order, that is, for something to happen—one thing follows another. When we put narrative discourse into play, it is to acknowledge and *live within* time—poetry cannot do this, epic cannot do this, and abstract prose cannot do this. Narrative discourse— novels, newspaper stories, Scripture, clinical conversations—is the lived evidence, the footprints, of our human progression through this element of time that encases us and that enables us to live and understand our lives.

All of the work of ethics is performed in the penumbra of time. If narrative is a response, leaving a trail, to temporality, then, in the Levinasian sense, responsibility to the other evokes the narrative, the series of queries and responses over time. In each conversation, as each participant in the discourse asks, is answered, and then continues, the trace of mutual discourse is recorded and told, and the task becomes to pass on the truth thereby exposed. This is the task bioethics shares with history, with literature, and with narrative. The ethics case, like the novel, is both paradigmatic and particular: our totality and our singularity are both celebrated and ruptured as the story—or the case—is told as an acknowledgment of and a resistance to time and mutability.

The paradox emerges here that time connotes, of course, death. And bioethics is the profession committed to facing death directly, calling out its name, and finally, unlike medicine, finding meaning in the lost places in the clinical world where death has established its dominion. Clinical and research medicine long ago erected death as the enemy, death as defeat. Through terror, perhaps, or through hubris, medicine endorsed the haunting illusion that it could conquer death. Despite the efforts of palliative care and hospice, attempts to understand and sometimes welcome death are marginalized and exert little influence on medicine's mainstream work—the big business of intensive care, clinical trials, and pharmaceutical and surgical intervention—all of which are predicated on finding the right triumphal ending for the narrative of illness.

For bioethics, death is the issue, the topic, the thing itself. Whether the actual question relates to futility, capacity, advance directives, abortion, cloning, stem cell research, or protection of human subjects, bioethics struggles to address the inevitability of death. The bioethicist—not the pathologist, not the geriatrician, not even the chaplain—is the holder of death's portfolio. At our best (and bioethics can fail terribly at this moment), bioethicists must create room among the living for the one who is dying so as to be alert to the idea of death. The task is to call attention to the limits of the triumphal arguments of medicine (*just one more treatment!*), to learn and to teach the knife edge of discernment, the narrative of closed borders and of tragic endings. The intersubjective certainty of death does not lose its terror, nor its countenance, but becomes familiar.[13] Hence, the query of the other is always, on some level, about also this: and I, too, will die?

Literary critic and philosopher Walter Benjamin, himself a contemporary of Levinas, and like Levinas writing during World War II in the situation of a European Jew in danger, while the logical positivist world of philosophy and medicine failed and fell around him, wrote that "[d]eath is the sanction of everything that the storyteller can tell. He has borrowed his authority from death."[14] In this he saw, with great creative precision, how the shadow of death is the warrant for most of human endeavor. Death, Levinas teaches, is the great unknown, the great mystery for which human beings have no light, no knowledge, and no preparation. "What is important about the approach of death is that at a certain moment we are no longer *able to be able*," Levinas writes in *Time and the Other*.[15] It is the frankness of the confrontation, the stillness and the slowness of the talk of ethics that underlies the theoretical issues at stake. What is taught, ultimately, in philosophy and in literature is the meaning of that "just life" that Levinas requires, a life continued as if bound to continue, which is possible only if one can continue to work in the lacunae of death. It is, perhaps, the central work of teachers of bioethics.[16]

DESIRING TEXTS

An aspect of narrative theory attracting much contemporary ferment is the desire inherent in the text. Not only the desire of individual characters in literary works, but the desires inherent in the telling itself, in the listening, and in the arrival at some mutual interpretation are being seen as pivotal engines powering us all toward and through one another's texts. The hunger to know the story's end joins with the propulsive drive to tell it to its end. All texts, by this gesture of literary theory, can be seen as the substrate for the appetites, reading and writing as mutual surrender, and textual activities as the erotics of penetration of text by reading, of reader by text.

But in clinical ethics, one both achieves and resists closure, thereby fulfilling the desire for completion and postponing its satisfaction. One achieves closure by transforming the real exchange into a fictive one as soon as the real exchange is complete—one changes the names and the details to obscure and protect the subject, one extrapolates from the actual case to make the moral point, and one becomes a character in the action ("The bioethicist agreed").[17] But one resists the closure as well. The bioethicist cannot know the story's ending and cannot control its ultimate outcome. The unruly other is, after all, not "ours," not, as Levinas notes, a stage in our moment of journey, but a member of a real family that continues and in whose life we may play, for all our self-importance, but a bit part. For the ethicist, the real case becomes the literature of bioethics and the actual is submerged in extrapolation. For the patient, who is the "object" of the narrative, the real is the way that her life, fundamentally altered by choices made, continues in time, while the literature of bioethics is unnecessary, and in the sense of the Mayan Indians, the lie.

The tension of achieving and resisting closure of the narrative is currently, perhaps, the most urgent open chapter in the cases of bioethics. This tension may explain why ethics as a discipline remains unsettled about theoretical moves toward narrative ethics or intersubjectivity. Conventional approaches to bioethics problems tend to limit their temporal horizons to that which can be seen during a hospitalization or a NICU stay. However, admitting narrative methods into the enterprise of bioethics encourages one to ask new questions—not only "Who among the family members should make the proxy decision?" but "And how has this family lived, afterwards, with what they have committed?"

Those aspects of the lives of patients and professionals brought into view by the deployment of narrative skill are uncontrollable, ever shifting, uncategorizeable. Like narrative does wherever it is released, narrative in bioethics supplants the formulaic and ordered with the singular and chaotic. As one's certainty and confidence (and sense of the blasé) plummet (never more to say, "We see this"), one opens one's eyes to an altogether new situation—not predictable, not probabilistically this or that, but altogether a first and only instance of what it is. Although we all are tempted to ask only questions that might be answerable, narrative methods—and the desires exposed by them—give us the heart to ask questions without answers, that is, questions that do not end. But there is more: as clinicians trained in philosophy and literary theory (your authors of even this chapter), we work as both moral actors who wish to be of some use in the clinic and as authors of the story of the case even as we live in the story of the case. We "tell" the case, and we explain the arguments and uncover the methods of the work of telling—the objective processes of how narrative "works." Yet we are also drawn to the emotive, subjective, and the unstable—hence the paradox of Descartes emerges even in the work of narrative theory.

NARRATIVE INTERPRETATION

Narrative ethics is intertextual, cross-coded to bioethicists' stories, to your (the reader's) story, to the patient's story, and to the larger canon of the moral imagination we share. In writing this article, we two colleagues have written of how we think a theory of narrative ethics can be understood philosophically (Zoloth) and textually (Charon) in a context of the clinical ethics we practice and teach and in light of a social and political history we share.

So Zoloth claims:[18] We live by stories, as narrative ethicists, and we see that the world has a series of tales needing resolutions; in some instantly recognizable way, this is true. We are told of an outside, factual world that is constructed for us first by narratives, long before we live in it as moral actors. By virtue of our stories, we know of emplotted knowledge, of retribution and revenge, and of choices and adventures. The sensory, empirical lifeworld of moral praxis can seem previously lived, reawakened into, because we can recall so strongly the knowledge of these tales. (One can think here of fairy tales we tell as children, long prior to the need for rescue by the Prince.) In this sense, both Platonic and talmudic,[19] all beings are born into a preknowledge that has merely been forgotten.[20]

These vaguely known, perhaps forgotten, but surely recognized stories surround us. Who can read of Gabriel in James Joyce's "The Dead" without a rich, earthy sense of unity with him, his dying demented aunt, his beloved wife who yet loves another? "Snow was general all over Ireland" cannot only refer to one country in the Northern Atlantic; the story's mournfulness and hope refer, surely, to "all the living and the dead."[21] Although chronologically impossible, I (Charon) cannot believe there was a time before I read those words. When I accompany mourning families after a death (and in the practice of a general internist, it happens regularly), I can honor the ravage and approximate the meaning of their grief, in part, through the thoughts of John Marcher in Henry James's "The Beast in the Jungle." "What had the man *had*, to make him by the loss of it so bleed and yet live?"[22] Events in our own lives recapitulate other events, not only when psychoanalytical transference replays relationships with parents but when one death recapitulates another, when one loss forces one to relive all the losses that led up to this freshest one. We would be bereft without this wealth of stories, without this echo of what is known and then forgotten, and without our human capacity to remember.

In a thoughtful essay about Greek epic narrative, literary scholar Erich Auerbach notes the difference between the detailed styles of Homer and the sparseness of the Hebrew narrative texts.[23] To Auerbach, the lacunae of the Hebrew texts create classic characters against whom we test ourselves. Stories are implied as suggestive type-scenes[24] that we recognize and repeat. The biblical master tale is necessarily one with gaps and losses. In this, it mimics the human narratives we glimpse in the lives of the patients and the health care providers we study. The gaps in the story then create the possibility of both intertextuality and of moral discourse. When no rule, duty, or motive is given, the moral activity is to argue and reason toward what they might be. Hence the interpretive community that surrounds all classic texts emerges to make stories *moral* stories, useful as well as aesthetically pleasing.

Who is the moral actor in narrative ethics? Who is the protagonist and what is her role? One can claim that ethics cases not only have the named players, plot devices, points of view, climaxes, and resolutions but that they have a story-space as well.[25] They are told as if we, the readers, inhabit them. In a complex and reflexive set of actions, readers write the text as they read. This is an exegetical method: this is how we read biblical texts, this is how we read the spare modern novel, this is how we read the glimpses of lives flashing by in popular culture. Its familiarity does not cancel out its ability to defamiliarize what we see, leading us to pause, as did William Carlos Williams in the wake of a patient in his office: "We catch a glimpse of something, from time to time, which shows us that a presence has just brushed past us, some rare thing—just when the smiling little Italian woman has left us. For a moment we are dazzled. What was that?"[26]

Intersubjectivity—this writing as we read—is perilous as it is generative. The text with the lacunae, the text with blank spaces, may indeed function, in an odd way, as a moral text when we first face it and then enter it interpretively. Kermode describes this feature of a text as "something irreducible, therefore perpetually to be interpreted; not secrets to be found out one by one, but Secrecy."[27] If we readers are agents, or more perilous still, if we think we come as the heroes in the ethics narrative—asked to judge and justify—then we are part of the consequential, responsible activity of ethics. We must duly answer, giving our own best approximation of the presence and the meaning of both the secrets and their cumulative secrecy, when the text asks, "And what do you think?"

Case stories, with their quirky spareness of detail, the way they have of possibly unfolding as *any* case in *any* clinic at *any* time would unfold, are understood by the reader like all type-scenes in literature—with stock characters and moral lessons we hope to understand and then tell. In our efforts to interpret the case story, we fill it in with what we know. Case stories function, then, by allowing us to infer much by design while requiring us to seek and uncover the moral possibilities and arguments. Kermode continues, "We glimpse the secrecy through the meshes of a text; this is divination, but what is divined is what is visible from our angle. It is a momentary radiance."[28] The possibility of permeability and inclusion enlivens the form and might lead us beyond narrative ethics toward an interruptive narrative, a multivocal conversation, taking into account what might be seen from all angles, in which there is overlapping assent, dissent, and always more telling.

As Levinas reminds us, reading a piece of literature differs from bearing witness to another real person in her need and with her power (to define us, to call on us, to reject our interpretation with her own). One creates a theoretical distance at some cost. And yet, says Charon, we gain in wisdom and insight by placing these two interpretive processes side by side.[29] Acts of clinical and bioethical interpretation can become more robust and more examined by exposing their sibling status with literary interpretation. We want ethicists to bring to bear on clinical texts—an ethics case, a progress note in a hospital chart, an operative report, or a conversation with a parent whose child has just died—the powers so rigorously and skillfully developed in years of reading literature. And, to bare the practical forearms of Charon's general internist self, identifying the kinship between ethics cases and literary stories *does* something of great value. It donates to us and to our trainees powerful, practical methods of developing, strengthening, and teaching these interpretive skills.

Finally, to place these sibling stories side by side reminds us that, as stories to be entered and lived through, clinical and ethical stories demand our most serious commitment and courage. All forms of reading—both epi-reading and graphi-reading—are called into play in these complex and perilous acts of interpretation. In formulating the literary notions of narrative ethics, Robert Eaglestone notes that "Levinas's approach to language allows both the ethical commitment to the world that the critical orientation of epi-reading demands and the acute concentration on the actual language of literary texts asked for by graphi-reading."[30] Levinas can lead us back to that bedside, no longer remaining vertical but sitting with the dying patient, on the risky diagonal, leaning forward, trying with all our might to enter his story-space, his realm of meaning. As ethicist, one struggles both to be aware of one's own interests and to understand beyond one's own cause, so as to achieve the humility and capacity to absorb and give voice to the cause of the other. One uses one's whole self—and is therefore irreplaceable—as an instrument to transduce the other's words and actions and plight into meaning.

CODA

These conversational and dialogic notes about narrative ethics became a midrashic, intertextual exploration of our discursive community. These are tentative notes, for we two ethicists draw from many places—the example of rabbinic culture, the literature of Henry James, the field of religion, the theory of narratology, and the practice of medicine. The conversation between us implies a Levinasian watching and listening third, who is the patient/subject/point of the story. It also implies a fourth—the reader of this chapter. We feel that we join with others in bioethics who struggle to be the place of the embrace of many and even contradicting ways of knowing and who struggle to find a common language, like a common truth claim, in order to fulfill our clinical duties.

We, Zoloth and Charon, are authors telling you, reader, a story we find credible, real, plausible, and this is affected by our lives as clinicians who need for our work to be of use, Charon being a doctor, Zoloth having been a nurse. But it is our training in literary scholarship and in philosophy that allows us to search for operative moral values in the arguments, to uncover the wheels and gears and pipes behind the work. In the process of so doing, we have found ourselves enacting both meanings of intersubjectivity—gazing from our separate personal and disciplinary angles of vision at narrative ethics to triangulate an interpretation and, in the process, reaching a communion of sorts through text and through practice. This mutuality, in the end, offers the fundamental ground for the discipline of narrative ethics.

NOTES

1. See Wayne Booth in this volume and in *The Company We Keep: An Ethics of Fiction* (Berkeley: University of California Press, 1988); Adam Zachary Newton, *Narrative Ethics* (Cambridge, MA: Harvard University Press, 1995); J. Hillis Miller, *The Ethics of Reading: Kant, de Man, Eliot, Trollope, James, and Benjamin* (New York: Columbia University Press, 1987); and Robert Eaglestone, *Ethical Criticism: Reading after Levinas* (Edinburgh: Edinburgh University Press, 1997), for recent studies of readers' and writers' duties toward one another.
2. Denis Donoghue, *Ferocious Alphabets* (Boston: Little Brown, 1981), 99.
3. Ibid., 43.
4. One thinks of the passing gunman in the Western story, "Shane."
5. Tod Chambers, *The Fiction of Bioethics: Cases as Literary* Texts (New York: Routledge, 1999).

6. René Descartes, "Discourse on the Method of Rightly Conducting the Reason and Seeking Truth in the Field of Science," in *Philosophical Essays* (New York: Bobbs-Merrill Company, 1964).

7. Barbara Herrnstein Smith, "Narrative Versions, Narrative Theories," in *On Narrative*, ed. W. J. T. Mitchell (Chicago: University of Chicago Press, 1981), 228. (Emphasis in original.)

8. Julia Kristeva, "Psychoanalysis and the Polis," in *The Politics of Interpretation*, ed. W.J.T. Mitchell (Chicago: University of Chicago Press, 1983), 86. In this essay, Kristeva explores the intersubjective dimensions of interpretation using Lacanian and Freudian psychoanalytic theories. Although not altogether salient to the project of bioethics, Kristeva's framework of semiotic desire generates helpful suggestions in examining the narrative situations of health care decision-making.

9. Robert Gibbs, introduction to *Why Ethics? Signs of Responsibility* (Princeton: Princeton University Press, 2000).

10. It must be noted here that since Heidegger, Levinas's teacher, was also, in a serious way, his betrayer (in that Heidegger was an early member of the Nazi Party and accepted the chancellorship of the university during the war years in Germany, while Levinas was a prisoner in a forced labor camp), Levinas also considered many aspects of his work dangerously wrong.

11. Emmanuel Levinas, *Outside the Subject*, trans. Michael B. Smith (Stanford University Press, 1994), 92. Subsequent page references to this work appear in parentheses in the text.

12. Frank Kermode, *The Sense of an Ending: Studies in the Theory of Fiction* (London: Oxford University Press, 1967), 45.

13. In the way of most literature, and with certainty the literature of the premodern text of the Talmud, which is the focus of Zoloth's research, and the work of James, which is the focus of Charon's.

14. Walter Benjamin, "The Storyteller," in *Illuminations*, ed. Hannah Arendt, trans. Harry Zohn (New York: Schocken Books, 1985), 94.

15. Emmanuel Levinas, *Time and the Other*, trans. Richard A. Cohen (Pittsburgh: Duquesne University Press, 1987), 74.

16. Who, like the nurses and the doctors, never stand outside the notion that death can be overcome with medicines and machines.

17. Chambers, *The Fiction of Bioethics*. In Chambers's work, we see how point of view alters the telling of the case.

18. Laurie Zoloth, "Making the Things of the World: Narrative Construction and the Project of Bioethics," *American Journal of Bioethics* 1, no. 1 (Winter 2001): 59–61.

19. Plato, *Five Dialogues*, trans. G. M. A. Grube (Indianapolis: Hackett Publishing, 1974).

20. The folk story of the Jewish world is like the Hellenistic one—that an infant learns Torah before birth, but just before he is born, the angel who teaches him places a finger to quiet his knowledge on his mouth, leaving a mark on his upper lip, the indentation under the nose—one's task is to relearn Torah in this sense, not to learn it.

21. James Joyce, "The Dead," in *Dubliners* (New York: Viking Press, 1968), 223–24.

22. Henry James, "The Beast in the Jungle," in *The Novels and Tales of Henry James: The New York Edition*, vol. 17 (New York: Charles Scribner's Sons, 1909), 124.

23. Erich Auerbach, *Mimesis*, trans. Willard R. Trask (Princeton: Princeton University Press, 1968).

24. Robert Alter, *The Art of Biblical Narrative* (New York: Basic Books, 1981).

25. See Seymour Chatman, *Story and Discourse: Narrative Structure in Fiction and Film* (Ithaca: Cornell University Press, 1978), 96–107, for a discussion of story-space as the stage or world within which fictive events are enacted.

26. William Carlos Williams, *The Autobiography of William Carlos Williams* (New York: New Directions, 1967), 360.

27. Frank Kermode, *The Genesis of Secrecy: On the Interpretation of Narrative* (Cambridge, MA: Harvard University Press, 1979), 143.

28. Ibid., 144.

29. Rita Charon, "The Life-Long Error, or John Marcher the Proleptic," in *Margins of Error: The Ethics of Mistakes in the Practice of Medicine*, ed. Susan B. Rubin and Laurie Zoloth (Hagerstown, MD: University Publishing Group, 2000), 37–57.

30. Robert Eaglestone, *Ethical Criticism: Reading after Levinas* (Edinburgh: Edinburgh University Press, 1997), 7.

PART II

NARRATIVE COMPONENTS OF BIOETHICS

CHAPTER 4

CONTEXT: BACKWARD, SIDEWAYS, AND FORWARD
HILDE LINDEMANN NELSON

I t is often assumed that, when ethicists work with cases, they are taking a narrative approach to clinical ethics. In this essay I argue that this is typically not true, at least for cases that find their way into print. In the commentary on the case, which is where the ethical analysis takes place, the commentator typically acts as a judge, applying lawlike principles deduced from one or several of the standing moral theories to the situation described in the case; so applied, the principles serve to prescribe the right course of conduct. Judging skillfully and well in accordance with some theory involves a consideration of the economic, cultural, class, gender, and religious contexts in which the participants operate, as these social contexts might have some bearing on which principles to select and how much relative importance to assign to conflicting principles. However, once the commentator has gotten hold of the correct principles and a rationale for ranking them, context is of no further interest. The commentator can now judge impartially what ought to be done in any similar set of circumstances.

After considering a case that has been treated in this way, I offer a *narrative* approach to the case. In a narrative approach, the social contexts are important, not because they guide the selection of the principles that will be used to resolve the case, but because of what they reveal about the identities of the participants: the religious, ethnic, gender, and other contexts in which a person lives her life contribute to her own and others' sense of who she is. How others see her crucially influences how they will respond to her, so it matters whether they get these contextual features right. While those who use the "juridical" method described above could in principle take the same view as narrativists of the moral importance of *social* contexts, only a narrative approach can work with the case's *temporal* context. Because juridical methods center on an ethical analysis of what is going on here, in the present moment, they tend to approach the morally troublesome situation as if it were atemporal. But understanding how we got "here" is crucial to the determination of where we might be able to go from here, and this is where narrative is indispensable. The story of how the participants of the case came to their present pass is precisely a story, as is the narrative of the best way to go on in the future. The backward-looking story is explanatory; the forward-looking story is action-guiding. Juridical approaches tend to move only sideways, considering context as it fleshes out the here and now. Because narrative approaches also move backward and forward, they are better suited to ethical reflection. They also, as I will explain, make of morality something quite different from what the standing theories have supposed it to be.

THE ORIGINAL CASE

Here is the case, entitled "Please Don't Tell," as it originally appeared in the *Hastings Center Report*:

> The patient, Carlos R., was a twenty-one-year-old Hispanic male who had suffered gunshot wounds to the abdomen in gang violence. He was uninsured. His stay in the hospital was somewhat shorter than might have been expected, but otherwise unremarkable. It was felt that he could safely complete his recovery at home. Carlos admitted to his attending physician that he was HIV-positive, which was confirmed.
>
> At discharge the attending physician recommended a daily home nursing visit for wound care. However, Medicaid would not fund this nursing visit because a caregiver lived at home who could provide this care, namely, the patient's twenty-two-year-old sister Consuela, who in fact was willing to accept this burden. Their mother had died almost ten years ago, and Consuela had been a mother to Carlos and their younger sister since then. Carlos had no objection to Consuela's providing this care, but he insisted absolutely that she was not to know his HIV status. He had always been on good terms with Consuela, but she did not know he was actively homosexual. His greatest fear, though, was that his father would learn of his homosexual orientation, which is generally looked upon with great disdain by Hispanics.
>
> Would Carlos's physician be morally justified in breaching patient confidentiality on the grounds that he had a "duty to warn"?[1]

As it stands, the case concerns the scope of a patient's right to medical confidentiality, which it frames as a question about the physician's obligations. The commentators accept this frame and answer the question accordingly: Leonard Fleck concludes that "the physician is morally obligated to respect that confidentiality," while Marcia Angell, reasoning differently, concludes that "the doctor should strongly encourage Carlos to tell his sister that he is HIV-infected or offer to do it for him" (p. 40).

Fleck, who is a formally trained moral philosopher, works out his answer by tacitly endorsing a principle: in the absence of excusing conditions, physicians have an absolute duty to respect their patients' confidentiality. He then considers the excusing conditions:

> (1) an imminent threat of serious and irreversible harm, (2) no alternative to averting that threat other than this breach of confidentiality, and (3) proportionality between the harm averted by this breach of confidentiality and the harm associated with such a breach. (P. 39)

Searching for each of these in turn in the facts of the case, he finds that none of them is present. He argues to his conclusion by a syllogism in the form of *modus ponens*: (a) if there are no excusing conditions, the physician's duty to protect his patient's privacy is absolute; (b) there are no excusing conditions; (c) therefore the physician's duty to protect his patient's privacy is absolute.

In his discussion of the excusing conditions, Fleck does take context into account. He reminds us of how difficult it is to become HIV-infected when doing wound care; he emphasizes that the dilemma arises because of Medicaid's rules for funding home nursing visits. These contextual features help him to establish likely outcomes of telling versus not telling so that he can assess the proportionality between the harm averted and the harm incurred in either scenario. However, once he has satisfied himself that none of the excusing conditions is met, context becomes irrelevant. It does not matter how the physician, his patient, or other third parties are situated. What is action-guiding is the principle and the absence of excusing conditions.

Whereas Fleck, concerned with both the results of an action and the duties that are owed to others, draws on a mixture of consequentialist and deontological moral theories to arrive at his conclusion, Angell, a physician by training, relies entirely on deontological theory. She speaks of Consuela's right to have information relevant to her decision to act as Carlos's nurse, the wrongfulness of deception regardless of the consequences, the special duties owed Consuela by a health care system that is "using her to avoid providing a service it would otherwise be responsible for" (p. 40). Even in her discussion of the risk of transmission from Carlos to Consuela, Angell seems less concerned with the harmful consequences to Consuela than with her right to decide whether the risk is acceptable to her. She agrees with Fleck that, absent excusing conditions, the physician's duty to protect his patient's privacy is absolute but finds that this principle cannot be applied in the instant case because there *are* excusing conditions. So she invokes another principle: respect for persons, which entails a right to self-determination, which cannot be exercised in the presence of force or fraud. Carlos may not manipulate Consuela by deceiving her, for that is to use her as a means to his ends solely. If this sounds Kantian, I mean it to, since in my view Angell has done a superb job of applying Kant's moral theory to the story of this brother and sister.

Like Fleck, Angell pays attention to context. She notes, for example, that the players are situated differently with respect to gender and implies that the power imbalances that accompany gender difference are morally relevant to the successful resolution of the case:

> I can't help feeling that this young woman has already been exploited by her family and that the health care system should not collude in doing so again. We are told that since she was twelve, she has acted as "mother" to a brother only one year younger, presumably simply because she is female, since she is no more a mother than he is. Now she is being asked to be a nurse, as well as a mother, again presumably because she is female. (P. 40)

But note that gender exploitation only compounds a wrong that would exist in any case, one that could be established to be a wrong even if we knew nothing about Consuela's gender. The principle of respect for persons, not considerations of context, is doing the lion's share of the moral work in this commentary.

RETELLING THE STORY SIDEWAYS AND BACKWARD

Let me now propose a different way of deliberating about this case, one that involves telling further stories. I contend that by pulling the case apart and retelling it so that it reveals the moral importance of contextual features that were originally played down or ignored, the deliberators can come to a better understanding of who the participants are and what the appropriate moral response to them might be. The backward-looking stories the deliberators tell about the participants have explanatory force: they supply the temporal setting that allows us to make sense of what the various actors are now doing.[2] The sideways stories also broaden our understanding of "now": they exhibit the effect of the various social contexts on the participants' present identities. Both sorts of stories show us more clearly who the participants are.[3]

Let me illustrate what I mean by supposing that "Please Don't Tell" is a case brought to the hospital ethics committee by the attending physician. I shall further suppose that while those with the most at stake ought ideally to be among the deliberators, Carlos's sister obviously cannot be present, since the question is precisely whether she is to learn of Carlos's infection. We shall suppose, therefore, that Carlos's social worker, who has talked to both Consuela and her father, was invited to the case presentation. Based on what she knows, she retells the case this way:

Consuela R., a twenty-two-year-old Hispanic woman, has been keeping house for her father, her brother Carlos, and her sister since her mother died when she was twelve. She is not a mother, any more than Carlos is, and has not tried to take her mother's place. She has merely tried to get dinner on the table and clean clothes in the closets and tend in general to everyone's domestic comfort. At first she tried to do this while going to school, but there was no one to stay with her sister when she was ill and Carlos was running with the gangs and her father couldn't seem to adjust to widowerhood, so she dropped out at sixteen and stayed home. Family life improved.

Now that her siblings are almost grown, Consuela would like to go back to school and learn business management. She earned her GED and has won a scholarship at a local college. She had just enrolled for the full course load the scholarship requires when Carlos was shot. Her father won't nurse the boy—he's too angry about Carlos's repeated troublemaking even to speak to him. And her sister has said many times she's not going to let the family eat her alive too. So it looks as if the wound care is up to Consuela, and that means part-time schooling, and that means giving up the scholarship. She wonders whether Medicaid would have paid for daily home nurse visits if she had already started living on campus, but she suspects Carlos would simply have gone without care. And that's not right. He's her brother and she loves him. He's worth what it's costing her.

Notice how the story told on Consuela's behalf picks up on the gendered context of the case and makes the same point about it that Angell's commentary does. Notice too, however, that where Angell's commentary uses gender only as a buttressing consideration, focusing mainly on what is owed to anyone who is in Consuela's position, the social worker's story lays out in some detail just who Consuela is. Knowing what she cares about, what she wants, and what her actions say about her character allows us to see more clearly what is at stake for Consuela if she tends her brother's wound. And because the story goes backward as well as sideways, we can also see the sorts of sacrifices she has already made and how these bear on the present moment. We were not so apt to notice, in the way the original story was told, that circumstances have forced Consuela to assume responsibilities that are too heavy for a child, and that these same circumstances have kept her from taking advantage of opportunities to make a better life for herself. The retold story, in fleshing out the temporal context of Consuela's life, allows us to see the ways in which not only her family but also the Medicaid system take advantage of her willingness to care for her father and siblings when no one else will do it. Once we see this, we are in a better position to decide whether Carlos is doing something wrong in insisting that she not be told he is HIV-positive.

The moral terms and general rules that can be brought to bear on Consuela's story need not be understood as inflexible laws. Instead, they can be regarded as markers of the moral relevance of certain features of the story: "Hasn't Consuela *sacrificed* enough?" "Isn't Medicaid being *unfair*?"[4] In the process of retelling the original story, the deliberators' understanding of these concepts may undergo a change. For example, the committee members may come to see that, even if she knew about her brother's seropositive status, Consuela's *consent* to care for the wound isn't a yes/no concept whose presence indicates that her care is voluntary and whose absence indicates that it is not. Rather, consent as we see it in the story seems to admit of degrees. Consuela consents, all right, but as the retold story indicates, she would consent more heartily to an arrangement that let her continue her formal education. Certain features of the retold story thus suggest ways of understanding the relevant moral ideas, and these ideas in turn may point to other previously neglected details of the story. The story is finished when the augmented context and its attendant moral concepts are in a state of equilibrium that allows the deliberators to see the situation from Consuela's point of view.

THE SECOND PASS

In taking the original story apart and retelling it to reveal the social and temporal contexts in which Consuela lives, the social worker has put important moral considerations on the table, but she has not gone far enough. If the committee members stop retelling the story here, they have stopped too soon. So let us suppose they take a second pass at retelling the story. We shall say that one of Carlos's nurses, who is a permanent member of the ethics committee, tells the next version, which she has pieced together from a few conversations she had with Carlos during his hospital stay:

> The patient, Carlos R., was a twenty-one-year-old, uninsured Hispanic male who had suffered gunshot wounds to the abdomen in gang violence and was HIV-positive. At discharge the attending physician recommended a daily home nursing visit for wound care. However, Medicaid would not fund this nursing visit because a caregiver lived at home who could provide this care, namely, the patient's twenty-two-year-old sister, Consuela.
>
> Carlos had no objection to Consuela's providing this care, but he insisted absolutely that she was not to know his HIV status. It's hard enough to be a gay man in any culture with a heterosexist bias, but in a Roman Catholic Hispanic culture, where sexual relations are moralized to a much greater degree than in secular society, Carlos feared with some justice that Consuela would stop seeing him as a brother and a man, and identify him primarily with his sexual activity. After all, even secular America talks about "actively gay," as if you were gay only when having sex. Carlos had already lost his mother at a time in his life when he was just starting to have to come to terms with his erotic indifference to women and interest in men, and because his father found it so hard to face life without his mother, Carlos had pretty much lost his father, too. What tenuous connection still remained would be snapped altogether if the old man knew his son was gay.
>
> Carlos was in desperate need of a family. That was why he had started running with his gang in the first place. He'd thought these were people who would be loyal to him and give him a sense of belonging somewhere. It hasn't worked out that way, however. The gang members abandoned him when he was shot and threatened to kill him if he revealed their identities. So Consuela, who has always been important to him and whom he loves very much, is really the only family he has left.

Because the original case is silent about a number of morally salient points, this retelling, like the previous one, has to augment as well as reassemble the original story's components in order to achieve an equilibrium of narrative particulars and moral terms. Note too that while the original story *looks* as if it is Carlos's story—which makes it odd that the nurse then retold it from Carlos's point of view—the case as initially presented is in fact a story about what the attending physician should do: it is told from within the ethical framework of physicians' responsibilities to patients. Most clinical cases are aimed at physicians and adopt the physician's perspective. For that reason, most of the narrative augmentation of the case moves backward and sideways to show relevant details about other characters in the story.

Like Consuela's story, this one enlarges the temporal context. It lets us see quite plainly where Carlos is coming from, which goes some distance toward explaining why he is so adamant about concealing the truth from his sister. The explanation suggests that his intention is not so much to use his sister as a means to his own ends solely as to safeguard a precious relationship, and in that way it opens up for reexamination Angell's earlier, juridical verdict. The story of where Carlos has been tells us something about who he is, as does the sideways view of the social context in which he lives his life.

CONSTRUCTING THE FORWARD-LOOKING STORY

We appear to have reached an impasse—on its face, not unlike the one Fleck and Angell arrived at in the pages of the *Report*. Fleck's analysis drives in one moral direction, Angell's in another; ditto for the stories of the social worker and the nurse. You tell your story, I tell mine. So what?

This is a question that is often raised about narrative approaches to ethics, mostly by skeptics who do not seem to notice the contradictory conclusions that can be derived from juridical approaches, which also invite a "So what?" response. When asked of narrative methods, however, the answer to that question is "Wait—we're not finished yet." When the case has been retold often enough to get a sense of who the participants are and what moral considerations ought to be brought to bear on them (and this might require a third or even a fourth pass, as the deliberators examine the father's and maybe even Medicaid's stories), it is time to tell the story forward. The moral deliberators do this by putting into equilibrium the details of all the previously told stories and the moral descriptions that are suggested by them. From their sense of how the narrative pieces shed light on one another, they then construct, together, the closing story of how best to go on from here.

In one scenario, the physician might arrange for a visiting nurse to come only every three or four days so that the family can afford what it costs to pay her, even if this means the nurse must provide suboptimal care. In another scenario, the home health agency agrees that the bill can be paid in small installments, to begin when Carlos is well enough to take a job. Various members of the committee contribute still other possibilities, revising and correcting the forward-looking story in light of the equilibrium that has already been achieved within each of the other stories.

The committee members' narrative activity is an attempt to identify or create a set of moral understandings that allow the participants to work out, together, what they should or must do now. Through the stories they tell, they seek a shared sense of what Carlos's predicament means for him, for Consuela, for the father, and for themselves as responsible professionals. The backward- and sideways-looking stories told in response to Carlos's troubling request are the medium through which they come to a kind of mutual moral intelligibility; the forward-looking story reflects that common comprehension.

If their forward-looking story is constructed *from here*, its assessment, as Bernard Williams reminds us, is necessarily *from there*.[5] The deliberators cannot know until the story plays itself out whether the possibilities they foresaw could actually be realized in the way that they anticipated. Something might turn up or have been overlooked that sends the story off in an unexpected direction, so that, in the event, there is cause for regret. Because the story is forward-looking, from here, it is somewhat indeterminate; from there, it might mean something morally that cannot now be seen.

And that is what I mean when I say that a narrative approach makes of morality a rather different sort of thing from what the standard moral theories have supposed it to be. On the juridical model, morality is a matter of solitary judges applying codified rules derived from comprehensive theories as criteria for assessing wrongdoing and making rational choices. This picture of morality represents it as a body of *knowledge*: the (solitary) moral philosopher's task is to construct, test, and refine covering laws that exhibit this knowledge, while the task of moral justification is carried out by the covering principles or procedures that make up the moral theory. The more one knows about the foundations of the theories, their content, their relative merits, and how they are to be applied to specific problems, the greater one's claim to ethical expertise.[6] And like other forms of expertise, moral knowledge is neither easily acquired nor competently wielded by amateurs.

In contrast, the narrative approach I have been describing is precisely one for amateurs. It sees morality as a continual interpersonal task of becoming and remaining mutually intelligible. In this view, morality is something we all do together, in actual moral communities whose members express themselves and influence others by appealing to mutually recognized values and use those same values to refine understanding, extend consensus, and eliminate conflict. The narratives we tell as we jointly and collectively decide what we ought to do help us make moral sense of our lives and create common expectations about which of us is responsible for what, to whom. Here, the authority for a moral intuition rests on its embeddedness in a shared form of moral life, while the basis for moral criticism lies in the tensions between, and the fissures within, the stories that circulate widely in the community. Anyone who doesn't share enough of the important intuitions is either a morally incompetent member of the moral community, or not of the community at all. "Mutual moral understanding," writes Margaret Urban Walker, "both presupposes and seeks a continuing common life. It requires a presumption in favor of accounting to others and trying to go on in shared terms."[7] It is *expressive* of who we are and hope to be; it is *collaborative* in that it posits, not a solitary judge, but a community of inquirers who need to construct ways of living well together. And because those constructions look forward, as well as backward and sideways, it is a view of morality in which the meaning of "now" is indeterminate and must wait on the event.

The juridical model has been under fire for quite some time, not only by narrativists but also by feminists, postmodernists, and other antitheorists of various stripes. Within bioethics, resistance to it can be seen in the many criticisms of "principlism," a juridical method popularized by Tom Beauchamp and James F. Childress in their widely influential *Principles of Biomedical Ethics*, now in its fourth edition. It is only recently, however, that criticisms of juridical approaches have been overtaken by the development of positive alternatives to those approaches. A body of theory, to which this essay attempts to contribute, is now beginning to form around one such alternative: the various kinds of moral uses to which narratives can be put. I have here been concerned with narrative methods of moral deliberation, but narratives arguably perform many other functions within the moral life. They cultivate our moral emotions and refine our moral perception; they make intelligible what we do and who we are; they teach us our responsibilities; they motivate, guide, and justify our actions; through them, we redefine ourselves. Accounts of *how* narratives function within morality are sorely needed, but the work has begun. For those of us who have become increasingly dissatisfied with the juridical model, the narrative turn in bioethics is welcome indeed. It will be most interesting to see where it takes us.

NOTES

1. Leonard Fleck and Marcia Angell, "Please Don't Tell," *Hastings Center Report* (November–December 1991): 39. Subsequent page references appear in parentheses in the text.
2. Alasdair MacIntryre, *After Virtue*, 2nd ed. (Notre Dame: University of Indiana Press, 1984), 211–12.
3. Annette Baier, *The Commons of the Mind* (Chicago: Open Court Press, 1997); Paul Benson, "Feminist Second Thoughts about Free Agency," *Hypatia* 5, no. 3 (Fall 1990): 47–64.
4. Margaret Urban Walker, "Keeping Moral Space Open: New Images of Ethics Consulting," *Hastings Center Report* (March–April 1993): 35.
5. Bernard Williams, "Moral Luck," in *Moral Luck: Philosophical Papers 1973–1980* (New York: Cambridge University Press, 1981), 20–39.
6. Walker, "Keeping Moral Space Open," 34.
7. Margaret Urban Walker, *Moral Understandings: A Feminist Study in Ethics* (New York: Routledge, 1998), 63.

CHAPTER 5

VOICE IN THE MEDICAL NARRATIVE
SUZANNE POIRIER

L iterary terms that describe the elements and functions of stories are
deceptively simple. As the other chapters in this section demonstrate,
concepts seemingly as straightforward as *plot, character,* or *context*
encompass a variety of choices on the part of the author and an equal variety of
consequences for the reader. *Voice* is no exception. In the pages that follow, I
examine the ways that three different literary scholars have discussed voice and
consider how their ideas can illuminate the way physicians tell stories to themselves and to other health professionals. Finally, I demonstrate how the limitations
of medicine's narrative voice can, in turn, limit discussion of the ethical and
human dimensions of medical care.

First, though, a brief reflection on grammar. *Voice* is both a noun and a verb.
As a noun, it is a mechanism for conveying the spoken word. As a verb, *voice*
implies agency, motivation. It always requires a direct object: "She voiced a concern"; "he voiced his agreement"; "they voiced their opinions." And, as a verb, *voice*
is attached to a subject, a person from whom the voicing emanates. *Voice* is thus
deliberate, purposeful, and personal. The term *disembodied voice,* by contrast,
usually refers to something supernatural or ethereal and is a cause for awe or fear,
precisely because it removes from our sight or direct perception the embodied,
identifiable agent.

Second, a brief consideration of a literary term related to voice: *point of view.*
The contrast of the visual with the vocal implies an immediate difference, but the
word *point* anchors sight to a particular person. The novelist Henry James probably stated it best in his preface to *Portrait of a Lady*:

> The house of fiction has in short not one window, but a million.... [A]t each of them
> stands a figure with a pair of eyes, or at least with a field-glass,... insuring to the per-
> son making use of it an impression distinct from every other. He and his neighbours
> are watching the same show, but one seeing more where the other sees less, one seeing
> black where the other sees white, one seeing big where the other sees small, one seeing
> coarse where the other sees fine.[1]

No one person can, literally, see the same thing as another. In medicine, this inevitable variation is acknowledged when a physician asks, for example, what the night nurse said about a patient's restlessness or various family members about their relationships with their dying mother.

Inherent in James's depiction of multiple viewers at different windows is the implication that what is seen by the eyes is also filtered through each individual's mind. James notes that each of these million windows "has been pierced, or is still pierceable ... by the need of the individual vision and by the pressure of the individual will."[2] Vision, as with voice, is mediated by an individual person who will interpret what is seen in terms of his or her own "needs" and "will." James describes the interpretive aspect of point of view as inevitable to and inseparable from human existence.

Voice, however, goes one step further in that it is an action rather than a perception. *Point of view* is a term that can only be used as a noun. Like point of view, voice draws upon the "needs" and "will" of the speaker, but it also involves a conscious turning outward, an expressiveness that will reveal (or, at times, attempt to conceal) point of view. Nurses reporting to the physician about a patient's restlessness will give information that they have been trained to observe and interpret as nurses, but they may give more or less information given their own work demands or even their feelings about the physician asking the question. Family members' willingness and thoroughness in discussing family relationships will obviously reflect unique relationships filtered through each person's emotions and anxiety in talking about these personal matters. Physicians who gather information from nurses and family members go on to assemble and report that information in ways that are useful to and have meaning for their professional work, but there is always the possibility that their personal perceptions will play into this reporting as well.

Although they are not fiction, many of these clinical reports take on a narrative form. Three of these forms are the case presentation, the team conference, and the medical record. The following three sections demonstrate how these standardized forms of medical narrative try—but ultimately fail—to make the professional voice the only one *voiced* by physicians. In recognizing the many facets of the narrative voice, physicians and bioethicists alike can tell their own and interpret others' stories more effectively.

STRUCTURE AND THE CASE PRESENTATION

The narrator of a novel or short story has many options in choosing a voice. A tale may be related by one of the characters in the story (Mark Twain's *Huckleberry Finn* is a familiar example), by an "outsider" who was purportedly told the events by one of the characters (as with the tenant Mr. Lockwood in Emily Brontë's

Wuthering Heights), or by any one of a variety of "omniscient" narrators who can see into the minds and hearts of various characters to various depths. The options are much more limited for the narrator of the case presentation. A large part of medical education is given to learning to perform and present the history and physical, differential diagnosis, and treatment plan in a particular sequence and in a particular style. The concise, nearly universal form of the case presentation is an important, necessary form in medical communication, but its standardization can mask the individuality that each narrative voice unavoidably contains.

Whose is the narrative voice of the case presentation during morning report, attending rounds, or grand rounds? Ostensibly, it is that of the medical student, resident, or attending physician who organizes and recounts the work done in the diagnosis and treatment of a patient. That work, however, was usually not solely done by the narrator. French literary theorist Gérard Genette's description of *narrative level* enables listeners to tease apart the variety of sources that culminate in the case presentation.[3] Genette observes that stories many have multiple tellings and that every retelling places the current narrator at a level further and further removed from the initial telling of the story. An example from literature is Margaret Atwood's *The Handmaid's Tale*, in which the narrator reports discovering a cache of audio tapes. Their transcription contains an account by a person who is relating not only events in her own life but events in others' lives as reported to her by them. In medicine, the case presentation contains information that is seldom the sole experience or purview of the teller's interaction with the patient. Moreover, that first *medical* narrative is itself a retelling and reinterpretation of the patient's narrative.

The narrative voice in the case presentation is thus both that of the individual telling the tale and a compilation of the voices of other, earlier narrators. Given this collective contribution to the case presentation, the most appropriate narrative voice might be a first-person plural *we* or a combination of first- and third-person *I* and *they*. In actuality, physicians are taught that the proper narrative voice is that of an immediate actor and participant who never says "I," "we," or "they." Most sentences are cast in a passive voice that erases the actual first-person narrator: "Upon examination, the patient was shown to have," for example. Two case presentations from morning report at my institution demonstrate the force and stricture of this form. (I will speak of myself in the first person on occasion in this chapter for the very reasons I criticize its absence in many medical narratives.)

In the first example, a first-year resident was recounting the events around the admission of a patient to his service the night before. A number of residents, several of whom were seated around the table, had been involved in the assessment of the patient and the decision to admit her. As he made his presentation, the resident acknowledged which person had discovered what information at different points in the long journey to diagnosis, at times turning to other residents to furnish details that they, and not he, had first observed. The chief of service was clearly unhappy with the presentation: its careful chronology and acknowledgment of others' contributions were not the voice of the standard case presentation. The resident was interrupted repeatedly by the chief, who insisted that information be given in the not-always-chronological order required by convention and cutting off the seemingly digressive, inclusive style of his narration. In a second instance, a senior resident, who was an acknowledged expert at both medical diagnosis and the form of the case presentation, deliberately flouted both the form and its voice: "I know I should tell you the lab results at this point, but it will ruin the story," she interjected at one point, to the amused tolerance of her supervisors. Their tolerance of *this* resident's unorthodox voice, in her knowing violation of the requisite form and its requisite voice, signaled their recognition that she had mastered both.

These stories demonstrate the deliberate creative process that moves a narrative voice in medicine from the first level of encounter with the patient through subsequent levels of examination, laboratory work, and oral presentation, passing along portions of the patient's story from one person, or group of people, to another. At this later level, the narrative voice is one that generally values conventional structure over dramatic effect.

Clearly, a systematic way to convey this ongoing story is necessary. This singular narrative voice, however, can become problematic as a patient's hospital stay continues. Over the days, sometimes weeks that follow, the patient will be examined and treated by numerous physicians, most of whom will also narrate the patient's course to others. Still, the narrative voice that tells the tale at rounds will remain virtually unchanged, implying a continuity and a consensus that may not truly exist. Presumably, anyone who "picks up the case" would tell a very similar story. Without the he-said, she-said of daily conversation or the quotes within quotes of fiction, the identity and context of each contributor is lost. What remains becomes a matter of record. When, for example, an early interviewer labels a patient simply a "poor historian," a vague term that could apply to any number of possibly transient conditions, that label follows the patient and is usually accepted without question as the story is passed along, the source and purported accuracy of its report buried under subsequent levels of narration.[4]

The deceptive seamlessness of the case presentation can make it difficult to raise—or even identify—ethical issues that may be a part of a patient's care. For example, in a monthly geriatrics conference, a resident told, in the standard voice of the case presentation, about a terminally ill man who had been placed on a ventilator when he came into the emergency room.[5] Attempts at weaning him had proved unsuccessful. What should be done? As the team members prodded for more information, they gradually learned that the presenting resident herself was the one who had helped intubate the man in the emergency room, unaware that he had a living will that would have prevented such an action. Now the man is writing notes to her saying, "I want to live," while the other residents are angry with her for having intubated him in the first place. When she tries to discuss his continued treatment, they cut her off, and when she pleads that his treatment should be considered in the light of his new desire to live, they refuse to consider her argument.

The resident's initial narrative voice, as she began to report the "case," was carefully modulated to present a sequence of medical information about a patient initially in crisis whose emergency treatment left him in a situation that was unfortunate but understandable. There was no place in the structure of the story to register this resident's role at the chaotic start of treatment, the growing tension in the intensive care unit as the patient remained on the ventilator, or the conflict she now feels between herself and her patient as well as between herself and her colleagues. "What I want to know is," she finally asked, her voice full of emotion, "did I do the right thing in the first place?" Of course she did, and the physician who headed the geriatric team was quick to reassure, explain, and comfort. She was finally able to voice—to people who would listen—the personal anguish and confusion that were not permitted voice in the professional case presentation.

This is not to say that no discussions of medical ethics occurred within this resident's medical team. Although the story she told suggests that any ethics discussion was scant and scantily informed, a case presentation was not needed for those discussions to occur on the hospital floor. What it does demonstrate is that, where the case presentation is the vehicle for discussing a patient's care, a narrative form that does not acknowledge the multileveled nature of its creation does not allow for a full exploration of ethical or personal dilemmas regarding that patient's care. As a narrative voice that strives for professional uniformity and objectivity by obscuring narrative levels and the diverse human input at each of those levels, the case presentation runs the risk of being a medically useful but ethically limited form.

DYNAMICS AND THE TEAM CONFERENCE

The geriatrics conference that I observed in the case described above was conducted as a teaching session for first-year residents in general internal medicine. The geriatrics team consisted of two physicians, a social worker, a nutritionist, a clinical pharmacist, and a nurse. In addition to the first-year residents, the social worker and nurses involved in the care of the patient under discussion usually attended as well. No treatment decisions were made, and the conference was not considered a consultation. Its sole purpose was to encourage young physicians to think of the wealth of factors that contribute to the health and illness of elderly people. Sometimes the greater part of a session focused on nutrition and ethnic food traditions, other times on the range of nursing facilities in Chicago and their differing qualifications for admission.

It was the personal inclination of the presiding physician to ask such questions as "How do you feel about this patient?" or "Would your job be easier if you didn't like this man so much?" When he retired, his successor continued to convene the conferences for another few months but changed them to become predominately medical in nature. The newly presiding physician clearly guided the hour, often lecturing about a particular illness and the latest scientific and clinical studies. Where the team's discussion under the former leadership incorporated multiple aspects of care, it now focused much more narrowly on biomedical concerns. Whether teams consist solely of members of one profession or represent a cross section of the health professions, most of them claim that their raison d'étre lies in the multiplicity of voices they bring to the table. This example demonstrates that the particular individuals composing the health care team influence it a great deal.

In their insistence on the importance of the multiple, diverse contributions of a range of practitioners, members of health care teams parallel Russian theorist Mikhail Bakhtin's celebration of the novel as an egalitarian site of multivocality.[6] Bakhtin dates the rise of the novel to coincide with the introduction of new people and competing worldviews into homogeneous communities. As communities became more diverse, through both the infusion of outsiders and the increased stratification of its own citizens, their languages also became more diverse with, for example, the dialects of foreign sailors or the formal writs of courts of law. These groups spoke *specialized languages*, and their words reflected the worldview or ideology of that specialty. Thus, the world became heteroglot, or multivocal, which the novelist embraces to create a *heteroglossia*, a cacophony of worldviews to be paraded before his or her readers. The novelist invites characters and narrators to talk together, debate, misunderstand each other, compromise, and disagree. This combination of voices broadens the novelist's thinking beyond the narrow range of his or her national or occupational realm and usually leads to a more complex view of the world.

This description of the many voices in the novel is relevant to the team conference in medical settings, in part for the way it reflects the many professional orientations that can inform decision-making. Sociologist Peggy Carey Best demonstrates this process in her analysis of a series of hospice team conferences about a patient who has recently been hospitalized.[7] Participants include hospital nurses, who are currently caring for the patient; a social worker, who helps to clarify sources of tension around the patient's care; a visiting nurse, who cares for the patient at home; a chaplain, who addresses some issues of ethics and patients' rights; a head nurse, who is coordinating the patient's hospital care; a nursing director, who is coordinating the patient's overall hospice care; and a medical director, officially in charge of decisions. The conferences, or "staffings" as they are called, are clearly multivocal, with each participant contributing a certain kind of knowledge and skill to planning the patient's care. The multivocality displayed in these staffings reflects part of the ideology of interprofessional teams, which holds that no single health profession can fully assess a patient's condition or needs.

How that information is processed and used, however, can vary. Although the physician, who must ultimately write most orders in a patient's chart, is usually the team leader, teams vary in the strictness of their hierarchy and the process by which a decision is made. If the different narrative voices provide data only, without any reflection on the meaning of that data or its relationship to other professionals' data, the conference lacks what Bakhtin calls *dialogism*. Dialogism goes beyond surface exchanges to create a new understanding of one's world. Bakhtin applied the concept to a novelist's ability to create a new vision from the many voices of a novel, but he went on to observe that it could occur in other narratives as well. Because all language is written or spoken in a social context and is intended to be communicated, it is rhetorical and invites dialogue, Bakhtin argues, whether in imaginary conversation between a novelist and reader or in a face-to-face conversation, such as the conference among health professionals described here. In such a process, the words that people use are loaded with all the cultural meanings they have accrued along with the personal and situational meaning invested by any one speaker. This *internal dialogization* of the word, says Bakhtin, "penetrate[s] the deep strata of discourse" where "individual differences and contradictions are enriched by social heteroglossia" (p. 284). For true dialogism to occur, whether in a team conference or in the mind of an individual reader, people must go beneath the words, to think about the worldviews represented by the words of the speaker or writer. Moreover, internal dialogization requires equal scrutiny of one's own words and worldviews.

Best's description of the hospice staffing includes this dialogism. She describes one instance in which the visiting nurse is helped by other team members to reexamine her evaluation of her patient, which has become perhaps overly influenced by her growing emotional involvement with her patient. In this instance, team members considered how the visiting nurse's story matched theirs, and when there appeared to be a dissonance, they—including the visiting nurse herself—looked beyond the words to her increasingly personal goals for and feelings about her patient. The dialogism among this array of specialized professionals allowed them to move beyond the overtly professional voice of one of their members and eventually to find a way to help not only the patient but also the distraught visiting nurse.

In this instance, the goals of the team included the welfare of its members. Members of the team not only attended to the professional voice of each member's story but searched as well for the personal voice that informed it. In contrast, several years ago I attended an ethics conference in which an intensive care team had earlier reached a consensus without dialogism, and, for reasons they could not explain, their work felt unresolved. The conference was called by the chief of the medical team, which included medical students, residents of every year, and the chief of the service. They wanted to discuss with the ethicists the withdrawal of treatment from a man who was in the final stages of a devastating illness, was no longer conscious, and who had left no written advance directives. His sister and mother, the latter on her way to Chicago from Virginia, had spoken in convincing, corroborating detail that their loved one had never wanted to end his life connected to medical machines. The nurses and therapists on the unit, along with the medical team, agreed that no possible improvement in his medical condition was possible and that his quality of life seemed negligible. The physicians reviewed this material with us calmly and compassionately. They presented medical and ethical arguments that seemed impeccable and carefully thought through. We could ask no questions that they had not considered, and they had no questions for us. They expressed no doubt about their decision. We complimented them on their process and their conclusions and wondered, in a slightly joking tone, why they had even called an ethics consultation.

"Oh, well, Alex over here," and the chief nodded his head to an L-shaped corner of the room that was beyond our sight, "thinks we're playing God." All heads turned to Alex, the only person in the room not at the table, sitting on the floor in his short white coat with his book bag at his feet. His eyes grew wide and he stammered, "No, I know, well, yes, this is best, but...but...it still seems, I don't know...." His voice trailed off. Noticing the short coat, one of us asked, "Are you a third- or fourth-year student?" "Third." This was early September. Alex had been in clinical clerkships for barely two months. "Have any of your patients died before now?" "This is the first."

We talked briefly about the pain of caring for a dying patient, particularly for the first time, but no one picked up on the conversation, and the consultation ended a few minutes later. Though I cannot speak to what conversations preceded this conference, the discomfort of most members of the team in acknowledging the medical student's anxiety or grief over a dying patient suggests that previous team conferences had not helped Alex grapple with his feelings. Dialogism among the team did not appear to have occurred, and where Alex was struggling with his own internal dialogism, he felt he was getting no help.

The dynamics of the narrative voices in health care teams, including bioethics teams, offer opportunities and challenges in the area of ethical decision-making. First, the multivocality of any team should be sought out, and both the professional and personal contexts of each narrative voice should be considered. Second, all teams should strive to foster truly dialogic conversations among all parties engaged in making that decision. Finally, if a bioethicist is called into a team situation, he or she should engage this dynamic of the group, and engage himself or herself in that process with them. Bakhtin's depiction of narrative voice is mutable, interactive, and culturally rooted, never static or monolithic. It reminds us in medicine of the importance of examining the complex power of the professional narrative voice to teach us about both patient and caregiver.

INDIVIDUAL VALUES AND THE MEDICAL CHART

In the preceding two sections the narrative voice of medicine has been criticized for its impersonal uniformity. Now, however, I suggest that there may be more of the personal narrative voice in the professional than many physicians might realize. U.S. literary scholar Wayne Booth argues that the novel is a text imbued with the values of its author, however difficult it may be for a reader to identify those values. He talks about the personal beliefs of the author, often subtly woven into the narration and containing "the inferable voice of the flesh-and-blood person for whom this telling is only one concentrated moment selected from the infinite complexities of 'real' life."[8] In medical narratives, so standardized and formulaic, it is hard to imagine where and how the "flesh-and-blood person" might peek through. One answer lies in the pressure, in medical as well as fictional narratives, of choosing, as quoted above, "concentrated moment[s] selected from the infinite complexities of 'real' life." The narrator in medicine must constantly edit his or her story as the daily work of medicine continues, retaining and removing selected pieces of information from the "infinite complexities" that accrue to medical care. In the interstices of these choices, ethically significant personal values are sometimes revealed.

One instructive example appears in the chart of a dying man during six weeks of his hospitalization, most of which he spent in a near vegetative state. His family, who was quite involved in his care, agreed that he would not want to be resuscitated should his heart stop beating. The attending physician noted in his chart that he would receive "comfort care" until he could be moved to a nursing home. This physician left shortly thereafter, and, when the patient developed a fever several days later, the new attending physician undertook an aggressive diagnostic evaluation, noting in the chart only the various tests and their increasingly dismal results. The social worker's chart entries frequently asked the physician to talk with the family, but there is no record of any such conversations. After a month, the next attending physician expressed concern over this treatment and asked to meet with the family. Subsequent entries in the chart spoke again of comfort care, no "aggressive" treatment, and the family's support of the DNR order.

The noticeably different entries in the chart by these three attending physicians, all in the appropriate form and language of medical charting, reveal different philosophies of treatment that are seemingly grounded more in personal values and feelings than in medical knowledge.[9] A curious side effect of the attending physicians' changing narrative voices in the chart is that the first-year resident, who was on the service throughout these three changes in attending staff, modified her charting voice to match that of each attending. Although this may have been a survival technique in the harried life of a house officer, readers guided by Booth's insistence that "the inferable voice" of the person writing in the physician's voice is present in that chart would have trouble knowing who this first-year resident is. Perhaps the resident's own narrative voice cannot appear in the medical chart until she is no longer answerable to attending physicians, but her changing narrative voice prompts the reader to wonder exactly what values she is learning and what she thinks about them.

Such a question is proper, according to Booth. Booth argues that it is the ethical responsibility of the reader or listener "to attempt to see how this tale works"—and that "[n]ot to do so...would be to deny the author's gambit" (p. 149). The "gambits" of the professional narrative voice of medicine are often subtle. The different medical orders of the three attending physicians were each, individually, perfectly coherent and medically reasonable. Only people who knew the possible options for treatment might identify different values behind the different orders. Some "gambits" may have more to do with things not said, such as the uncanny sense of agreement initially conveyed in the ethics consultation about withdrawing treatment (in the preceding section) or the shifting themes of the resident's charting.

Not only in written but also in oral language, the flesh-and-blood author can be perceived. One gambit, employed by a second-year resident in an ethics conference in internal medicine, was the repetition of one word in his case presentation, a word not usually occurring in the medical lexicon of my institution. The resident was reporting on a patient with unremitting, increasing pain, whose source could not be determined although it appeared to be real enough. The patient also had a past history of damaging tobacco and drug use but had not been using either for some time, "apparently," the resident said. "Apparently" was repeated throughout the chronological story of the patient's hospitalization, which included a variety of attempts to treat the pain, test the patient's veracity, and follow diagnostic dead ends. "Apparently" nothing helped this "apparently" agonized patient. Further questions revealed that the senior resident, not present at the conference, had announced her decision to resign from this patient's care.

Although the resident spoke nothing of this decision in his formal presentation, his obvious use of this nonclinical word invited questions from respondents, who then teased out this story of frustration and anger. The students and residents gathered for the conference accepted a directive that "physicians do not abandon their patients," but they were unwilling to talk about the anger most of them felt and how, together, they might find ways to help themselves and their patient. To some extent, the presenter's narrative gambit, while not an invitation to a dialogic conversation about the dilemma, served as means of communicating his unhappiness to listeners who recognized his break in narrative convention. In its own way this single word generated a knowing and, one supposes, a sympathetic response among the listeners, but no one felt invited to turn the conversation toward finding a solution to the problem.

CONCLUSION

The examples used throughout this paper should not be taken as an indictment of all medical-ethical communication and decision-making. More often than not, the participants in ethics conferences and the writers of medical reports struggle to understand the nature of the patients they treat and the problems they all face. Also, in the vast majority of instances, the professional narrative voice of medicine serves the needs of patients and physicians admirably. The forms of medical narration should not be jettisoned, but they can be used more effectively if the tellers of and listeners to medical stories become more astute as to how the forms and elements of narrative shape the stories.

The professional narrative voice of medicine has been carefully designed to present medical and some psychosocial information efficiently and consistently. When people with different values or moral beliefs are among the many tellers and retellers of the medical tale, however, this prescribed voice is not equipped to accommodate the ethical or emotional complexity that often results. The inability of many ethics discussions to address the personal values or feelings that often undergird ethical dilemmas suggests that the desire to deny or bury the personal voice under a formalized professional one may limit expression that is valuable to the conversation of bioethics.

The armor of a specialized narrative voice in medicine is strong but not impermeable. It can be pierced by the astute listener who exercises attention, creativity, and self-consciousness. The listener must detect the many narrative levels in the various forms of medical stories and be alert for lacunae or inconsistencies as a patient's story is taken up by another physician and then another. The listener must find ways to ask questions that will encourage a storyteller to speak in a voice that goes beyond the professional narrative voice in which she or he has been so carefully schooled. And because this new voice, a more deliberate melding of personal and professional, will take the now vulnerable storyteller into untried and often threatening narrative ventures, the listener must be prepared to explore those stories with their teller in order to learn what this narrative voice can teach them both.

NOTES

1. Henry James, preface to *The Portrait of a Lady*, in *The Novels and Tales of Henry James: The New York Edition*, vol. 3 (New York: Charles Scribner's Sons, 1909), x–xi.
2. Ibid., x.
3. Gérard Genette, *Narrative Discourse: An Essay in Method*, trans. Jane E. Lewin (Ithaca: Cornell University Press, 1980), 227–31.
4. I thank my colleague Daniel Brauner for this observation.
5. In this and all other case examples that I give, details of patients' and health professionals' identities, conditions, and sometimes gender have been changed as much as possible. For a fuller discussion of this case conference, see Suzanne Poirier and Daniel J. Brauner, "Ethics and the Daily Language of Medical Discourse," *Hastings Center Report* (August–September 1988): 5–9.
6. Mikhail M. Bakhtin, "From the Prehistory of Novelistic Discourse" and "Discourse in the Novel," in *The Dialogic Imagination: Four Essays*, ed. Michael Holquist, trans. Carol Emerson and Michael Holquist (Austin: University of Texas Press, 1981), 41–83, 259–422. Subsequent page references to this work appear in parentheses in the text.
7. Peggy Carey Best, "Making Hospice Work: Collaborative Storytelling in Family-Care Conferences," *Literature and Medicine* 13 (1994): 93–123.
8. Wayne C. Booth, "Who Is Responsible in Ethical Criticism, and for What," in *The Company We Keep: An Ethics of Fiction* (Berkeley: University of California Press, 1988), 125. Subsequent page references to this work appear in parentheses in the text.
9. For a fuller discussion of this chart, see Suzanne Poirier and Daniel J. Brauner, "The Voices of the Medical Record," *Theoretical Medicine* 11 (1990): 29–39.

CHAPTER 6

TIME AND ETHICS
RITA CHARON

The earthly predicament predicates time. Animate beings and inanimate things age. Be they made of metal or of wood or of stone or of flesh, objects wear. Chemical, biological, planetary, cosmological, and emotional reactions occur in steps. Causality connotes sequence. Communication requires tense. Simultaneity is nearly unattainable. Timelessness is unbearable.

Although one *is* oneself over the course of a lifespan, one adapts, matures, does one thing in the face of having done another. In an essay about his own liver transplantation, American poet Richard McCann mourns the loss of his earlier bodies. "I could still recall the body I'd had when I was ten, the body in which I carried what I called 'myself.'...I could recall the body I'd had, nervous and tentative, when I first made love at seventeen. But these bodies were gone, as was the body into which I'd been born, these bodies I'd called 'mine' without hesitation, intact and separate and entire."[1] He realizes, of course, and helps his reader to likewise realize, that his own "self" is permanent despite the profound and innumerable transformations of age. Literary critic Percy Lubbock writes that Tolstoy "is the master of the changes of age in a human being. Under his hand young men and women grow older, cease to be young...with the noiseless regularity of life; their mutability never hides their sameness, their consistency shows and endures through their disintegration."[2] Human beings are held aloft in a time that "flows," unaware except at the bidding of illness or of art how beholden we are to the buoyancy of our medium; without its invisible hand, we sink like stones into death.

Unlike the propositional thinking of moral philosophy, the epiphanic awareness of some forms of poetry, or the synchronic (that is to say, simultaneous or all-at-once) perception of the visual arts, the kind of human knowledge expressible through and experienced in narrative gives voice and shape to time. E. M. Forster states boldly that "what the story does is to narrate the life in time" and that, in the novel at least, "the allegiance to time is imperative."[3] Chapter 7 of *The Magic Mountain* opens with the observation that "time is the medium of narration, as it is the medium of life."[4] "Time," thinks protagonist Hans Castorp, "brings things to pass."[5] Because word follows word in temporally meaningful patterns in narrative forms of expression, inevitably inscribing and enacting the conditions of temporality, narrative forms of knowledge and expression seem a natural part of the human equipment. The first genre that humans speak is, after all, narrative prose. Developing narrative competence enables a baby to tell of himself or herself in so-called crib narratives, equips the youngster to absorb family myths and bedtime tales that reveal where he or she comes from, and authorizes the adult to acknowledge and envision the stories that constitute the self.[6] As philosopher Paul Ricoeur writes, "[B]etween the activity of narrating a story and the temporal character of human experience there exists a correlation that is not merely accidental but that presents a transcultural form of necessity. To put it another way, *time becomes human to the extent that it is articulated through a narrative mode, and narrative attains its full meaning when it becomes a condition of temporal existence.*"[7]

No act stands outside of temporal relation with what came before or will next occur, its meaning evolving retrospectively and prospectively. Although some so-called truths—the carbon atom has six protons, red and blue make purple—might appear timeless, they are easily seen as determined by or bounded by the mathematical time connoted by counting or the sequentiality of actions required for creation. The word *narrate* itself combines roots meaning "to count" and "to tell," literary critic Ross Chambers reminds us, suggesting that one "might thus imagine narrative as the counting out, item by item, of the contents of accumulated wisdom."[8] Hence, narrative contains, almost like a repository or reliquary, aspects of human knowledge and experience that can, once stored—and *storied*—be drawn on again and again.

The body, including its brain, works diachronically—that is to say, within time—and must submit to the limits inherent in the condition of temporality. Biological organisms live *in* their bodies—governed by the timed cycles of cell division, enzymatic reaction, synaptic release of transmitters, electrical rhythms of cardiac muscle and brain wakefulness. Individual organisms cannot exist outside of those times, except when, for example, in vitro fertilization enables a post-menopausal woman to bear a child or a cardiac defibrillator trumps a sick heart's beat. Such commonplace idioms as "stages of life" or "phases of development" point to the saturation by time of each organism's living. The difference between the pupa and the butterfly is no more vast than the difference between the adolescent and the young adult. No doubt brains have memory but so do livers and hearts. How, except by being endowed with memory, would a liver know the time has come to synthesize more 3-hydroxy-3-methylglutaryl-coenzyme A reductase? How would a heart know, beat by beat, what RR interval to repeat? The body never stands still—much as any plastic surgeon would like to convince you it can—and the body never forgets where it has been.

The body might have to bow to time, but what about the self? There is perhaps no concept more vexed, more combated, more often redefined, or more vital to consider than that of the subject, self, or identity. This is not the place to rehearse the Cartesian *cogito*, the Nietzchean logic of the fictional self, philosophical ideals of autonomy, Western theories of individualism, phenomenology's efforts to harmonize subject and object, or deconstruction's death of the self. The self, whatever that concept might have meant in the past or might mean in the future, can provisionally be thought of now as the "site" (the "address," if you will) for the singular individual—within his or her body, history, and conscious-ness—at the nexus of social, political, linguistic, geographic, aesthetic, cultural, genetic, gendered, familial forces that act on and are influenced by the self that will emerge from its moment.

This self is inscribed in its stories, and time is its obligatory coauthor. Students of autobiography have come to join cognitive psychologists, psychoana-lysts, phenomenologists, and neurobiologists, among others, in believing that the self cannot be created—or even found—independent of narrative activities. That is to say, the self emerges when the infant begins to tell stories about himself or herself, and the self develops through the intricacies of telling and retelling those self stories.[9] Such self-revealing and self-creating narratings weave out of, into, against, and toward time.

A hallmark of fiction, at least since modernism, is the ease with which tem-poral frames shift. The reader meets Virginia Woolf's Mrs. Dalloway in the pre-sent-day preparations for her party, is then brought back fifty years—by means of the sensory reminder of the squeak of a door hinge—to girlhood summers at Bournton, to slightly more recent adolescent loves and losses, and then forward again into the recent past of World War I. As Ricoeur notes about *Mrs. Dalloway*, "the narrator...offer[s] the reader an armful of temporal experiences to share."[10] Nurse Hana in Michael Ondaatje's *The English Patient* discovers the meaning of her care for her burned patient by traveling achronologically—and bringing the sometimes perplexed reader with her—through recent World War II experiences, memories of her father forty years ago in Toronto, and the recent loss of her mother—while the English patient himself performs equally high-wire time travel. In *So Long, See You Tomorrow*, William Maxwell enacts the boyhood losses of a now elderly analysand through a dazzling counterpoint of temporal juxtapo-sitions in several characters' lives. The governing image of the novel is a house being built with only the two-by-four frame visible, and the reader gradually real-izes that the transparency of one room to the other signifies the elusive trans-parency of past, present, and future.

Why do Woolf and Ondaatje and Maxwell tax their readers' comprehension by adopting complex and dense temporal scaffolding? The novelists adopt meth-ods from life. One does not make meaning chronologically. In performing any act of personal reflection, one does not think systematically about Monday and then move to Tuesday. Instead, one is bombarded by thoughts, sensations, revelations, and states of awareness that trigger one another through flashes of association or metaphor. We learn who we are backwards and forwards, early memories taking on sense only in the light of far later occurrences and contemporary situations interpretable only in the web of time.

Illness and its counterpart, health, are by definition time-bound.[11] Under-standing the meanings and significances of disease and recovery is as unruly an interpretive activity as is reading Woolf, Ondaatje, and Maxwell, demanding equally nimble navigation in time. The events of bioethics, too, are enacted in the flow of time, in part because of their intimate relations to those of the body and in part because of their intimate relations to those of living a life. The events of medicine and of bioethics must be captured in narrative in order to be beheld in their organic, timeful whole. When literary scholar Georg Lukács writes of the novel, he could be writing of our consultation notes: "Only prose can ... encompass the suffering and the laurels, the struggle and the crown, with equal power; only its unfettered plasticity and its non-rhythmic rigor can, with equal power, embrace the fetters and the freedom, the given heaviness and the conquered lightness of a world henceforth immanently radiant with found meaning."[12] What bioethics may gain by its current turn toward narrative knowledge and practice is a robust means of being accountable to time, answerable to its power, and cognizant of its hand.

I heard a case on a visit to a distant department of medicine. The intern presented me the case of a sixty-six-year-old woman recently admitted to the medical service with end-stage non-small-cell lung cancer. She had been diagnosed about three years ago, declined surgery and chemotherapy, choosing instead nutritional therapy and prayer to treat her illness. She had done unexpectedly well in the interim. However, at the time of hospital admission, she had developed abdominal swelling, tender nodes in the axilla, and shortness of breath that confined her to her bed.

As I heard this story during morning rounds, I imagined how on earth these young doctors and their senior attending physicians responded to the case. Were they enraged that the patient had postponed potentially helpful *real* treatment? Were they shocked that anyone would dare to substitute carrot juice for a lobectomy? Did they begrudge help to the patient now, after she had denied them the chance to cure? So I asked them to specify exactly what they went through as they listened to the case, and many members of the team gave voice to their anger that she had accepted Western medicine only when it was clearly too late for it to work, their frustration that a relatively young woman was needlessly dying, and their impulse to blame the patient for her current predicament.

I then asked them to imagine the state the patient was in now. We developed a robust "differential diagnosis": the patient was gravely ashamed to have waited so long before accepting Western medicine; she turned to us in anger and resentment once trapped by the progress of her disease; she felt guilty at this perhaps avoidable health crisis; she felt her relatively asymptomatic last three years had vindicated the methods of her natural healers; she was proud to have done so well with her alternative treatment and was now ready to accept another approach with serenity. Although we did not know which of these hypotheses approximated the patient's state of mind, at least we felt we had tried to imagine some of the infinite number of possibilities, and we felt prepared to try to inhabit the world of the story.

We met the patient in her hospital room. She described a courageous, faith-saturated journey through her ordeal shared with family, church members, and those who prayed for her from afar, her work in the family grocery store connecting her to a supportive community. She had made what any of us would call a reasonable choice, based on how poorly friends of hers had done with conventional cancer treatment and how the behavior of Western doctors had, if anything, added to her friends' suffering. She sensed great victory, not *over* the oncologist and Western medicine, but in her own physical stamina and resiliency as the disease, in fact, seemed to subside. That she had been relatively well these three years without surgery and chemotherapy she took as a sign that God was answering her prayers.

All of us surrounding her in her hospital bed felt nourished by her faith, disarmed by her honesty and gratitude, and unanimously on her side as she sought our help. We realized that, had she accepted surgery and chemotherapy at the time of diagnosis, we would have taken credit for her "good" years, and so we were willing to grant credit to her other avenues of health.

This example demonstrates how deeply embedded in time are the events and choices faced by ethicists and health professionals. What is at stake here is not diagnosis or treatment but rather such questions as "Is it too late? Why didn't she come to us earlier? Isn't she too young to die of this disease?" What we caregivers had to do in order to be present with the patient, respectful of her choices, and therefore useful to her is to travel in time with her, not only back to the time of the disease's onset but, really, back to the springs of her faith and the start of her own life journey guided by her beliefs and traditions. Our usefulness to the patient and her family was also to be measured in our capacity to envision and enter a future with them, not necessarily one scripted by us but one shaped by decisions made long ago.

Like in a novel or short story, the temporal dimensions of this story include the discourse-time, that is, the time it took the intern to tell me about our patient and the story-time, which here was not only the three years since diagnosis but the sixty-six years of the patient's life.[13] The relations between discourse-time and story-time are consequential, for the narrative *now* is established in discourse-time and alters events in story-time, whether or not the narrator realizes it. The teller gathers up great power in the course of establishing the beginning, middle, and end of his or her story, thereby framing the reader's or listener's temporal horizons. In the words of Paul Goodman, "[I]n the beginning anything is possible; in the middle things become probable; in the ending everything is necessary."[14] Even though the listener thinks that all the teller gives is the facts, in fact the listener is *acted upon* by all the teller's choices—the temporal dimensions as well as other aspects of style—making the listener far more indebted to the teller's worldview and deep notions of causality and consequence than it may seem. The intern started his story in the conference room with "This is the first X General Hospital admission for this sixty-six-year-old woman with untreated non-small-cell lung cancer who presents with shortness of breath," and seemed satisfied to report on the events of the last three years, except perhaps for the descriptor "nonsmoker, no exposure to asbestos." I had to gently renegotiate with him the beginning of our story, pushing the horizon back and back until, at the patient's bedside, we began prior to her birth.

Gérard Genette devotes over half of his masterful narratological study *Narrative Discourse: An Essay on Method* to inspecting narrative time.[15] He distinguishes three dimensions of time for discussion: order, duration, and frequency. Any moviegoer or novel-reader knows that the order of events in a representation can be altered, giving rise to flashbacks, flashforwards, and the like. Any teller, even the most naïve, will use such temporal dislocators as "before that" or "up until then," signaling through natural narrative behavior that order is not given but chosen.

Duration is a feature of storytelling that lives deep within the relationship between teller and listener. Only our greatest tellers of stories—Leo Tolstoy, Thomas Mann, Marcel Proust, maybe the writer of Genesis—have the power to convey the duration of actions and to re-create, in the reader, a sense of immersion in the tempo, rhythms, and course of time of the lives represented. Duration dramatically distinguishes the discourse-time from story-time in medical stories, because the professionals' view—including the bioethicist's—of "what happens" is restricted to such medically salient events as courses of chemotherapy or perioperative periods, while the patient is left to endure all that time between relapses and remissions, between taking the CT scan and learning its results, between the morning and evening dose of pain medicine.

Once the temporal horizon, order, and duration have been established, the teller can exercise surprise and suspense, two extraordinarily important elements of time-keeping in stories. The very enterprise being undertaken in medical or bioethical stories embroils tellers and listeners in the *expectations* inherent in such functions as predicting, prognosing, and beating the odds.[16] What any intern or health professional or bioethicist must resist, however, is the constriction of expectation to fit the universe of what one can oneself dream up. That is to say, we must all insist that the patient himself or herself will be able to surprise us far more fundamentally than we ever think.

Now, with expectations put into motion, the teller or listener of a medical or bioethical story is poised to enter the intersubjective space, that place where present meets the future. Whether I listen to an intern presenting at morning report or interview a relative stranger on visiting professor rounds, I am entering a relation with another, and it is within the intersubjective space created between us or among us that meaning occurs. Philosopher Emmanuel Levinas brings us to the point when he writes, "The situation of the face-to-face would be the very accomplishment of time; the encroachment of the present on the future is not the feat of the subject alone, but the intersubjective relationship. The condition of time lies in the relationship between humans, or in history."[17] And so, with whatever preparation we have made for entering the life space of another, we open ourselves, again and forever for the first time, to the experience of time.

Mrs. Castelli entered my care when her internist retired. (The patient upon whom this description is based has read—and has written parts of—this account. She has given me permission to publish it here. Nonetheless, I have changed her name and identifying features of this clinical description to protect her privacy.)

Then in her midsixties, she had been treated for mild hypertension, osteoarthritis, and anxiety that had been managed with Valium. Early on in our relationship, we tried to get to the bottom of her anxiety, and, in the course of learning the sources of her fears, I learned of her life. She had been involved in two abusive marriages, had raised three children on her own, protecting them from harm, and had managed to work full-time as a social worker in the public school system. Once we replaced the Valium with intensive supportive psychotherapy, the patient found the courage to divorce her second husband.

As I often do, I wrote down what I heard Mrs. Castelli say about what led up to her current clinical situation and asked her to read it so that she could correct or affirm my accruing understanding of her situation.

> She loved her house. She loved the flowering pear tree in the yard. This wood frame, three-story structure off Pelham Parkway contained her only memories of adult happiness. She could stand at the door of what she still called the "girls' room," imagining her two little ones preparing for bed, talkative as kids get near bedtime, their Catholic school navy jumpers and white blouses ironed for the next morning and hanging on the closet door. She could still gaze at Tom's collection of maps and atlases, fingered with imagined trips to the North Pole, the Equator, or the moon. And, for whatever reasons, she felt comforted by reminders of her and Frank's happiness too. The kitchen cabinets they had bought cheap and installed themselves. The basement they refinished as a playroom for the children and then a workshop for Frank. The attic they insulated as a study room when Gladys was at City. The house held within itself the history of a loving and normal family. That it had gone wrong Ellen knew but still could not understand or explain. Despite its ultimate failure, she wanted to be faithful to its undeniable successes.
>
> Ellen had hired the lawyer, signed the complainant papers, and paid the court fees. Frank did nothing. He did not contest. He did not object. He let the divorce happen to him, much as he had let his marriage and family happen to him. He did not move out of the house but remained, an unwelcome tenant.
>
> Then, after the divorce, Frank got lung cancer. A cigarette smoker since his teens, he had been in more or less good health until 1994, when he got progressively short of breath, developed chest pain, and lost a great deal of weight. Dr. Nadelson said the tumor was quite advanced when they first x-rayed it, too big for an operation. All they could do, the doctor said, was chemotherapy to limit the spread and radiation to treat the pain and breathlessness.
>
> It was just before Frank's cancer showed itself that Ellen had found the courage to move out of their house. After years of indecision and anxiety and paralysis and Valium, she had finally forced herself to act on her own behalf. She had rented an apartment for herself in New Rochelle, convenient to her job but far enough from the house to be in a separate place. Despite her great and wordless love for her house on Buhre Avenue, she moved her belongings out. Her daughters and her son helped her; her husband's unchanging passive rage helped her; mostly her own native sense that she deserved better changed her. The time had come for her to move.
>
> After they met with the oncologist and the radiotherapist and made a plan, Ellen made uncharacteristically quick decisions: Frank would move into the new apartment with her, and her son Tom and his wife and kids could have the house. Everybody fol-

lowed her orders: Frank moved in, Tom and his family took the house, and she found herself in the terrifying and satisfying position of being in charge.

Mrs. Castelli cared for Frank in her little apartment, giving over her newly-won independence for the sake of her husband. The chemotherapy and radiation sickened him; he refused hospitalization and gave himself up to his ex-wife's care. Although I had written about this stage, too, of Mrs. Castelli's life, she herself wrote a far more powerful description:

> Frank became weaker and sicker with every day that passed. The oxygen machine became something that would help him live and at the same time lulled me to sleep on the overburdened nights. Before I knew it he was hoping to die, and would ask that I pray for him. We could cry together but for different reasons. I cried for what could have been. When he could no longer breathe with the machine at home, he was hospitalized for evaluation. During this time he fell and broke his pelvis; the pain was unbearable and the morphine drip was started. It was now the beginning of the end. He never thanked me for the care. I guess he just sort of expected it, like everything I had done throughout our marriage. I still feel all mixed up because I know that I felt love for him very deeply. I miss him now more than ever, even though he was never my companion. For the first time in my life I feel alone. I feel cheated out of so many things. I know that I did the right thing although it leaves many people puzzled. I visit his gravesite and I still cry, not really knowing why. I guess the question will always be there.

This document traces, and perhaps enacts, authentic ethical activity. Not by coincidence but by necessity, both parts of it are narrated with a heightened awareness of time passing, both creating and demanding change. The ethical nodes in this story are not the ethicists' dilemmas, although some of our routine concerns regarding end-of-life care and familial duty do surface. Instead, the ethical dilemmas are the patient's own. Mrs. Castelli is involved in the pure ethics of examining her own life, plumbing her capacity to fulfill her duties toward others, and evaluating the beneficence of her actions. That this occurs in the internist's office is no surprise. Where else do persons typically get the chance to review their actions and to evaluate their life choices?

Since she suffered the loss of her husband, she has continued to make examined life choices. When her daughter moved back to New York from California and wanted to live in the house on Buhre Avenue, Mrs. Castelli mediated the complex demands and conflicting entitlements of her kids. She struggled to find a way to be fair to all three, denying no one, endorsing no one as more deserving than the others. She has taken seriously her own desires for a new life and is facing all the turmoil of making her way in the world as a newly single, more than middle-aged woman. Only in this retrospect is she able to appreciate her strengths—her remarkable capacity to care for others, to offer direction to others, to help others to find the meaning of their lives. By virtue of her deeply ethical actions, she lives a life of overwhelming inspiration, of authenticity, of bravery, and daring hope.

That I, as her internist, have had the privilege to witness and accompany her through the decades has taught me fundamental lessons, not about bioethics, but about the ethics of life.

These two courageous women facing illness and life choices are the most powerful messengers I can invoke to convey the gifts and essential temporality of narrative ethics. Literary scholar Kenneth Burke suggests the ethical nature of these women's narrativity: "By the ethical dimension, I have in mind the ways in which, through language, we express our characters, whether or not we intend to do so.... [W]e could say that language reflects the 'personal equations' by which each person is different from any one else, a unique combination of experiences and judgments. Thus there is a sense in which...each poet speaks his own dialect."[18] Our task as doctors, nurses, therapists, and ethicists is to learn each patient's personal language in its tenses, its images, its silences, and its tensions. That these narratives must unfold in time grants us the time to hear them, to provisionally understand them, and perhaps, thereby, to be of help.

NOTES

1. Richard McCann, "The Resurrectionist," in *Best American Essays of 2000* (Boston: Houghton Mifflin, 2000), 101.

2. Percy Lubbock, *The Craft of Fiction* (New York: Jonathan Cape and Harrison Smith, 1931), 51.

3. E. M. Forster, *Aspects of the Novel* (San Diego: Harcourt Brace Jovanovich, 1985), 29.

4. Thomas Mann, *The Magic Mountain [Der Zauberberg]*, trans. H. T. Lowe-Porter (New York: Vintage/Random House, 1969), 541.

5. Ibid., 544.

6. See Paul John Eakin, *How Our Lives Become Stories: Making Selves* (Ithaca: Cornell University Press, 1999), for an accessible and resourceful review and forecast of contemporary understandings of the intimate relation between narrative actions and the creation of the self.

7. Paul Ricoeur, *Time and Narrative*, vol. 1, trans. Kathleen McLaughlin and David Pellauer (Chicago: University of Chicago Press, 1984), 52. (Emphasis in original.)

8. Ross Chambers, "Narrative and the Imaginary: A Review of Gilbert Durand's *The Anthropological Structures of the Imaginary*," *Narrative* 9 (2001): 101.

9. Jerome Bruner, *Making Stories: Law, Literature, Self* (New York: Farrar, Straus, and Giroux, 2000).

10. Paul Ricoeur, *Time and Narrative*, vol. 2, trans. Kathleen McLaughlin and David Pellauer (Chicago: University of Chicago Press, 1985), 102.

11. Rita Charon, "Medicine, the Novel, and the Passage of Time," *Annals of Internal Medicine* 132 (2000): 63–68.

12. Georg Lukács, *The Theory of the Novel: A Historico-philosophical Essay on the Forms of Great Epic Literature*, trans. Anna Bostock (Cambridge, MA: MIT Press, 1971), 58–59.

13. See Seymour Chatman, *Story and Discourse: Narrative Structure in Fiction and Film* (Ithaca: Cornell University Press, 1978), 62–84, for a discussion of this important distinction.

14. Paul Goodman, *The Structure of Literature* (Chicago: University of Chicago Press, 1954), 14, quoted by Chatman, *Story and Discourse*, 46.

15. Gérard Genette, *Narrative Discourse: An Essay in Method*, trans. Jane Lewin (Ithaca: Cornell University Press, 1980), 33–160.

16. See Jerome Bruner, chapter 1 in this volume.

17. Emmanuel Levinas, *Time and the Other*, trans. Richard A. Cohen (Pittsburgh: Duquesne University Press, 1987), 79.

18. Kenneth Burke, *Language as Symbolic Action: Essays on Life, Literature, and Method* (Berkeley: University of California Press, 1966), 28.

CHAPTER 7

THE IDEA OF CHARACTER
ANNE HUNSAKER HAWKINS

A young junior resident in medicine, Michael Lewis, is asked by his attending physician, Dr. Peter Sharp, to go and see Mr. Pearsall, a fifty-five-year-old policeman with cancer of the esophagus, and get him to sign on to a promising clinical trial. Dr. Sharp tells him that Mr. Pearsall, who has been hospitalized repeatedly over the past year for treatment of his cancer, may well refuse the treatment out of hand. But the particular treatment protocol, Dr. Sharp tells him, is this patient's only chance at survival—moreover it seems a real advance in the treatment of this form of cancer and may well result in saving countless lives. Michael goes into the hospital room and finds that Mr. Pearsall is sleeping. At first he feels a flash of impatience—it's late in the day and he's already put in twelve hours on this shift. As soon as he can consent Mr. Pearsall, he can go home. But as he looks at the sleeping man, noticing how wasted and pale he looks, his impatience subsides. Michael sits down: he's been on his feet for hours. His gaze wanders to the pictures and cards on the bedside table. Wife, kids, and esophageal cancer: what rotten luck, he thinks. He closes his eyes briefly, reflecting on his amazing good fortune in being assigned to Dr. Sharp, a brilliant oncologist who is running a huge research protocol involving a new drug for just this kind of cancer. If Michael can impress Dr. Sharp, his career could really take off. Dr. Sharp reminds him a little of his own father, now dead—a brilliant geologist who had made major contributions to environmental science.

Mr. Pearsall coughs, and Michael opens his eyes to find that the patient is awake. He goes over to the bedside, introduces himself, explains the protocol, and tells Mr. Pearsall that he has a consent form for him to sign. Mr. Pearsall shakes his head. He won't sign: he tells Michael he's sick of tests, treatments, hospitalizations. Michael talks with him some more, persuasively, praising the study and ending with the very words he heard Dr. Sharp use, "It's your only chance." After more questions from Mr. Pearsall and vague promises or evasive replies on the part of Michael, Mr. Pearsall agrees. "You're the first person here I can trust," he says as he signs the document.

As Michael walks out of the hospital, he reflects on Protocol 907. He is uneasy. He knows that it's too soon to determine whether or not patients will be helped by this new combination of drugs; he has also seen how very sick they get as a result of treatment. He didn't lie to Mr. Pearsall about these side effects, because Mr. Pearsall didn't ask.

The next day, after a troubled night's sleep, he returns to the ward. When Dr. Sharp learns that Michael was able to consent the refractory Mr. Pearsall, he gives his resident a nod of approval. Michael looks in on Mr. Pearsall as he makes his rounds. They talk, and Mr. Pearsall confides in him—talking about his family, his memories, his hopes. Michael remains uneasy. Mr. Pearsall reaches over and grabs Michael's arm, looking intently into his eyes: "You know, it just feels so good to know there's somebody here I can trust. You're a fine young man, you remind me of my son—he was killed on the job. Freak accident." Tears well in his eyes as he says this, and he turns away to the window. Michael finds, to his surprise, that he is deeply moved by this confidence and the gesture that accompanies it. He reflects with bitterness on the glib promises he made to Mr. Pearsall last night. Then he leaves the room.

Michael returns about twenty minutes later, carrying Mr. Pearsall's chart. He opens it and tears out several pages at the end, handing them to Mr. Pearsall, who looks up in surprise. "This is what you signed last night," Michael explains. "I didn't really tell you the truth. I'm sorry. I can't promise you that this treatment will help you because it's too soon to know anything. And I know you're tired of tests and treatments that make you sick—the truth is that the patients I've seen tend to get really sick on this protocol. I'm sorry. I was wrong to talk you into signing this."

How can we best understand what transpires in this story? Michael feels enormous respect for Dr. Sharp: How can he present Dr. Sharp's protocol without trying, even if only unconsciously, to influence the patient's decision? But the focus here is not on the degree to which Michael did or did not follow the rules for seeking informed consent; rather, the issue is why he did what he did, what made him change midstream, and what he learned from this experience. Michael tries to reproduce Dr. Sharp's utilitarian approach, but it doesn't work—or, rather, it does work, but then Michael feels that he has betrayed his patient and to some extent himself in the process. Why does Michael feel this? Why does he go back to Mr. Pearsall, apologize, and tear up the consent form? Largely, it is his feelings as well as his developing relationship with Mr. Pearsall that instruct him how to behave. Observe the many emotions that are present—some partly concealed—under the surface of this narrative: respect for Dr. Sharp (and admiration of his own scientist-father), fatigue, pity; then discomfort, compassion, and shame. Michael does not turn to the principles of biomedical ethics—beneficence, nonmaleficence, justice, and respect for patient autonomy—to clarify his thinking. Even if he did, these principles require interpretation, and interpretation would take him right back to personal feelings, biases, and agendas.

The case I have outlined bears a striking resemblance to a text that at first seems utterly remote—Sophocles' *Philoctetes*. The resemblance is close because I have manufactured it, "translating" the ancient Greek drama into a medical episode that we might see dramatized on television's *ER*. Mr. Pearsall is a modern version of the Greek hero Philoctetes, who suffers from an agonizing wound that won't heal; Dr. Sharp is like Odysseus, and Michael is like Neoptolemus. Both are stories about moral learning and the moral development that is an inevitable consequence of moral learning. Both involve a process that transcends the narrow utilitarianism of Dr. Sharp or Odysseus, not by resorting to moral rules and principles but by emotional learning and respecting relationships with immediate others. Structurally, both involve a turning point in the action—a *peripeteia*—that is a result of moral recognition. In Greek tragedy, the idea of character is bound up with these dramatic processes of reversal and recognition.

The *Philoctetes* belongs to the kind of tragedy Aristotle calls "ethical" (my translation) precisely because it centers on character.[1] The link between character and *ethos* becomes only too obvious when we reflect that our modern word *ethics* has the same root as *ethos*, the Greek word for character. Ethics, today, tends to be thought of as a branch of philosophy. But Greek tragic poetry has an equally strong and even older claim to the transmission of ethical wisdom. In ancient Greece, it was the poets and the tragedians, rather than the philosophers, who were regarded as the primary teachers of ethics. So Homer could be called the "educator of Hellas,"[2] and his successors, the tragic poets, could be regarded as sources of moral guidance: "Little boys have teachers who instruct them," writes Aristophanes in *The Frogs*, "but when they grow up, the poets become their teachers."[3] Indeed, before Plato, there seems to have been no distinction between a "philosophical" and a "literary" presentation of human problems; similarly, there was then no sense of difference between a text devoted to the pursuit of truth and a text whose purpose was entertainment.

Still, one might ask, "Isn't Greek tragedy, with its masks, its stylized speeches, and its chorus, too different and too remote from today's world to have any relevance to contemporary medical ethical thinking and practice?" This may seem to be so, but it is also true that we can often understand aspects of our own culture better by looking at another. As Bernard Williams observes, "The demands of the modern world on ethical thought are unprecedented, and the ideas of rationality embodied in most contemporary moral philosophy cannot meet them; but some extension of ancient thought, greatly modified, might be able to do so."[4] A play like the *Philoctetes* gives us a very different picture of biomedical ethics than the idea of ethical decision-making as the application of abstract rules to a depersonalized problem—or as an encounter between "noncompliance" or "incompetence" in a hospital gown and a principle like "beneficence" or "respect for patient autonomy" wearing a white coat. The key elements missing from this formula are the character of the patient and the character of the doctor as well as the human interaction between them. The *Philoctetes*, as I hope to show, offers us a compelling model of ethical decision-making, of the factors that shape character and lead to right decisions between persons—in this case between doctor and patient—at the intersection of their life histories.

Character (*ethos*) in Greek drama is a specifically moral concept. The Greeks made a distinction between a person's inborn nature, which they called *phusis*, and his or her character, or *ethos*. *Phusis* is a more or less static concept; it is those qualities or capacities that we were born with. *Ethos*, though, is capable of development; it is confirmed, strengthened, and defined through the choices that we make—for better or worse. *Ethos* is not the vivid outward traits that make for personality, nor an individual's distinctive psychological makeup, nor the inner, often unconscious drives of the psyche—aspects of character that we expect, seek, and admire in modern literature. Of course, personages like Medea and Oedipus suffice to remind us that figures in Greek tragic drama do not necessarily lack colorful personality or psychological complexity and depth. However, what is essential to the action of Greek tragedy is the *ethoi* of these heroes and heroines, and *ethos* is determined by the choices evident in what they do or say. In a play (or in life) today, we might expect character to dictate the nature of the action. Put differently, we do what we do because of who we are; but for the Greeks—Aristotle especially—character tends to be seen as a function of the choices we make and the actions that result from those choices. As Aristotle observes, "Character is that which reveals moral purpose—that is . . . what kind of thing an agent chooses or rejects."[5]

Philoctetes, perhaps more than any other of the tragedies of Sophocles, is a quintessentially ethical play: it is concerned with moral issues, it focuses on the development of character through moral decision-making, it enlists the devices of tragedy as articulated by Aristotle to show us how moral learning takes place. Not only, then, does the play enhance our understanding of certain ethical problems; it also illuminates the very process by which we identify, analyze, and resolve those problems.

There are two claims regarding the way the *Philoctetes* demonstrates moral learning. The first concerns the utility of the emotions. The play demonstrates that our emotional responses function as heuristic tools for evaluating an ethical dilemma and coming to a decision as to what action seems best. In this, the play is in sharp contrast to the emphasis on systematic analytical reasoning advocated by Plato—an emphasis reflected today in versions of biomedical ethics based on analytic philosophy. Generally, today, we cultivate in ourselves and expect of others a dispassionate, objective, rational frame of mind when confronted with ethical issues. This play, however, shows emotional responsiveness as necessary in reaching sound moral decisions, and thus for the development of *ethos*. As Martha Nussbaum observes, "the passional reaction, the suffering, [is] itself a piece of practical recognition or perception."[6]

In this emphasis on emotion as central to moral character, the *Philoctetes* is very close to Aristotelian moral theory. Throughout Book II of the *Ethics*, Aristotle almost always links action with feeling (*praxeis kai pathe*) in discussing the virtues. Aristotle's theory of the virtues, argues L. A. Kosman, is "a theory not only of how to *act* well but also of how to *feel* well; for the moral virtues are states of character that enable a person to exhibit the right kinds of emotions as well as the right kinds of actions."[7] Moral character is thus manifest not only in what we do but also in what we feel. Of course, this is not to claim value for emotionality in and of itself; rather, Greek drama subjects emotions to intellectual and moral scrutiny. As Charles Segal observes, in Greek tragedy powerful emotional reactions are "pulled into the orbit of moral questioning and raised to a level of poetical and sometimes philosophical reformulation."[8]

The second claim is that the moral life cannot be conceived apart from one's relationships with others—a claim that contrasts to modern notions of the self as an isolated unit and that challenges the notion of the moral life as guided by abstract ideas, rules, and principles. An individual's "character" in Greek tragedy is a function of relationships with immediate others. Perhaps this is the reason why in this play, which may well be the most "ethical" of ethical tragedies, there are two heroes. The play does not center on either Philoctetes or Neoptolemus; instead, it is about the interaction between them and the interplay of both with Odysseus. By extension, the moral life is based on responses and obligations to other human beings.

The story of the play is as follows. The Greek warrior Philoctetes, who suffers from an extremely painful and repulsive foot wound, has been abandoned for years on a deserted island. Philoctetes suffers not only from the wound in his foot but also from his prolonged social isolation. The Greeks have learned that they need Philoctetes and his bow if they are to conquer Troy. The shrewd and seasoned warrior Odysseus and the youthful Neoptolemus arrive on the island with a mission: to bring Philoctetes—with his bow—back to the fighting at Troy, a return that will result in the healing of his wound. Acting on the advice of the older Odysseus, Neoptolemus gains Philoctetes' trust, then tricks him into handing over the bow, without which he is helpless. Just at this point in the play Philoctetes succumbs to an agonizing seizure of pain, which Neoptolemus witnesses. Neoptolemus is deeply moved by the extent of this man's suffering. Gradually, he realizes that he has wronged Philoctetes and violated his own moral nature in deceiving him. After a period of moral confusion, Neoptolemus tries to undo his wrong, returning the bow to Philoctetes and at the same time trying to persuade him that it is in his best interest to return with them to Troy.

The characters of Odysseus and Neoptolemus represent rival ethical positions. At the beginning of the play, both Odysseus and Neoptolemus are, in a sense, in agreement: they want Philoctetes to return to Troy, an action that will bring about victory for the Greeks and healing for him. Each suggests a different strategy: Neoptolemus wants to persuade Philoctetes; Odysseus insists they use trickery. As the play develops, the difference between the two widens. This widening difference turns on emotion: on the one hand there is Odysseus's willingness to sacrifice everything for a larger purpose, a stance made easier by his inability to feel pity for the obstinate Philoctetes; and on the other hand there is Neoptolemus's unease with using deceit as well as his growing sense of compassion for the suffering Philoctetes. Odysseus's relationship with Philoctetes remains instrumental: he is willing to manipulate him in order to achieve a larger goal, the conquest of Troy. Neoptolemus's relationship with Philoctetes develops, eventually, into one of reciprocity—what the Greeks called *philia*.

Whereas Neoptolemus is ensnared by reason and argument, he is rehabilitated principally by his feelings. The first part of the play depicts Neoptolemus's growing sense of compassion for Philoctetes (often voiced by the chorus), even as he pursues Odysseus's plan of deceit. It is compassion that brings him to an empathic understanding of Philoctetes' suffering, and it is through shame that he is able to acknowledge that he has wronged Philoctetes. The emotional forces that make for right decisions are deployed in what seems a hierarchical pattern: shame is directed toward the self; pity toward another. The play thus explores the relationship between private states of feeling and interpersonal relations: *ethos* for Neoptolemus is a function both of emotional learning and of honoring his obligations to persons (as opposed to principles or abstractions).

The conflict between his emotions and the Odyssean plan comes to a head during the scene of *pathos*, Philoctetes' agonizing seizure, which Neoptolemus witnesses. This is in every way a central scene, coming precisely at the midpoint of the play and introducing a line of thinking and feeling that leads to the play's turning point. Just after Neoptolemus asks to hold the bow and Philoctetes consents, Philoctetes invites him to come with him into the cave—into his inner experience. His sickness, he says, seeks to have Neoptolemus "stand by him."[9] This scene offers an icon of tragedy itself. Neoptolemus is a spectator to Philoctetes' agony as we are spectators to the paradigmatic suffering of the Greek tragic stage. Philoctetes bursts forth in a long, rhythmic cry—*pappapai papapa* (776)—that is inarticulate and untranslatable. He asks Neoptolemus if he understands his pain, and Neoptolemus replies that the pain is *deinos* (755)—a word meaning "terrible" but also "strange" or "wonderful." That Neoptolemus uses the right word for Philoctetes' suffering is an important marker in a moral development that gradually converts affective response into intellectual insight. Later on, Neoptolemus admits to a "terrible pity" (965; *oiktos deinos*) for Philoctetes. To refer to an emotion like pity as *deinos* is to acknowledge its compelling quality and to recognize its moral authority over one's choices and actions.

Neoptolemus's recognition that he has committed a moral wrong leads to the play's turning point, some four hundred lines later, as he gives the bow back to Philoctetes. The act is based on a decision that exemplifies the kind of purposeful decision, or *prohairesis*, that for Aristotle constitutes moral character.[10] Such decisions blend the intellectual and the emotional—here, Neoptolemus's understanding that his behavior has been wrong and the intense and angry sense of shame that accompanies it. Recognition (*anagnorisis*) and reversal (*peripeteia*), those classic Aristotelian elements of Greek tragedy, are here a part of the moral trajectory of the play. Neoptolemus's moral *anagnorisis* thus includes a recognition of the wrong he has done as well as the choice he must make to set it right. It is this choice that produces the play's reversal. Returning the bow is thus a characterizing act: who Neoptolemus is—his *ethos*—is a function of this act.

But Neoptolemus's gesture does not end the play or resolve the conflict in its plot. Though Sophocles emphasizes the role of feeling in Neoptolemus's moral education, he also shows, in his characterization of Philoctetes, that feeling alone is not a reliable guide to right action. The danger of emotion, in and of itself, is shown in the play's other hero, Philoctetes. In contrast to Odysseus, who seems devoid of feeling for either his youthful ally or his sick adversary, Philoctetes is full of passionate feelings. Indeed it is this passion that makes him obstinate in his refusal to return to Troy. It takes an act of divine intervention, a deus ex machina, to resolve the action of the play, as the divine Heracles descends to order Philoctetes to give up his anger, accept healing, and return to his heroic task.

When we turn back from classical tragedy to the fictional drama of Michael Lewis and Mr. Pearsall, our excursion through Sophocles and Aristotle helps us recognize certain important issues in medical ethics. Clearly, this young resident, like Neoptolemus, starts with the right *phusis*, an innate and natural disposition toward the good. We can surmise that like so many young medical students and physicians, he has become a doctor in order to help others. But this generalized benevolence is not enough: *phusis* needs to develop into *ethos* through repeated ethical choices and decisions. Michael's original decision could be justified on grounds of beneficence, since Michael is promoting research that may help many others while at the same time promoting the interests of his own patient. But this general principle is wrong for this particular patient. Mr. Pearsall trusts Michael, and Michael cannot promise that the research protocol will help him. Michael must thus recognize and then reverse his mistaken course of action. As in Sophocles' play, this episode of recognition and reversal results from feeling, from a sympathy that combines response to Mr. Pearsall's suffering and awareness of Mr. Pearsall as a particular and individual human being. Right choice turns out not to be the application of a general and abstract principle but a decision that derives from feelings of shame and pity conjoined to *philia*—the interactive relationship between persons who happen to be doctor and patient.

Though my story stops when Michael hands back the document and apologizes, this is in no way a conclusive ending. Similarly, Michael's character is not finalized through this act of recognition and reversal. Character, or *ethos*, whether in a modern ethics case or an ancient Greek tragedy, is a narrative construct in an ongoing story that continues beyond the play's ending. It may be that, like Philoctetes, Mr. Pearsall will finally join the research protocol or that, like Neoptolemus later on in life (when he slaughters King Priam), Michael will with some other patient make an ethical mistake that contradicts the *ethos* he seems to have achieved here. Precisely because *ethos* is always evolving, it must always be provisional—even precarious.

Were my story a Greek tragedy, I could provide a fit conclusion, one that would neatly resolve the tangled plot, by writing in an episode involving a deus ex machina. But, of course, the conventions of the ethics case do not allow for such an ending. Moreover, in ordinary life—whether today or in fifth-century Greece—there are few acts of divine intervention as spectacular, as conclusive, and, some would say, as factitious as the epiphanies at the end of Greek tragedies. Perhaps, though, the very artifice of its deus ex machina ending suggests an analogy between the *Philoctetes* and the genre of the ethics case. Tod Chambers argues persuasively that bioethics cases often refuse closure: instead, they end either with a question or by requiring the reader to rewrite the last part of the narrative and come up with a "better" conclusion.[11] Either way, this is a strategy with a purpose: the reader is expected to use some particular moral theory or moral paradigm to bring about a sense of finality. Perhaps the high artifice of a deus ex machina resolution in a Greek play is similar to the importation of some moral theory or the application of moral principles to "solve" an ethics case.

Rather, moral decision-making in medicine is a complicated process of using all of one's faculties—intellect, emotions, and imagination—to evaluate a particular situation and determine how to act. Central to such an evaluation is a keen awareness of the particular individual involved as well as an appreciation for the relationship between oneself and that particular individual. Also important is the capacity for self-awareness, which makes it possible to realize when one has made a wrong decision, correct the error as much as possible, and learn from the experience. The dilemma, and often the agony, of personal choice can never be obviated, even after a lifetime of practice in making difficult decisions. This seems to me the exercise of ethical medicine.

NOTES

1. Aristotle, "The Poetics," in *The Basic Works of Aristotle*, ed. Richard McKeon (New York: Random House, 1941), 1455b33–56a2.
2. Plato, *The Republic*, trans. Francis MacDonald Cornford (London: Oxford University Press, 1941), l. 10.606e.
3. Aristophanes, *The Frogs*, trans. Richmond Lattimore (Ann Arbor: University of Michigan Press, 1962), ll. 1063–66.
4. Bernard Williams, *Ethics and the Limits of Philosophy* (Cambridge, MA: Harvard University Press, 1985), vii.
5. Aristotle, "The Poetics," 1450b8–9.
6. Martha C. Nussbaum, *The Fragility of Goodness: Luck and Ethics in Greek Tragedy and Philosophy* (Cambridge: Cambridge University Press, 1986), 45.
7. L. A. Kosman, "Being Properly Affected: Virtues and Feelings in Aristotle's Ethics," in *Essays on Aristotle's Ethics*, ed. Amélie Oksenberg Rorty (Berkeley: University of California Press, 1980), 105.
8. Charles Segal, *Interpreting Greek Tragedy: Myth, Poetry, Text* (Cambridge, MA: Harvard University Press, 1981), 348–49.
9. Sophocles, *Philoctetes*, ed. and trans. Hugh Lloyd-Jones, Loeb Classical Library ed. (Cambridge, MA: Harvard University Press, 1994), 675. Subsequent references to this work appear in parentheses in the text.
10. Aristotle, "The Nicomachean Ethics," in The *Basic Works of Aristotle*, ed. Richard McKeon (New York: Random House, 1941), 111b3–12a17.
11. Tod Chambers, *The Fiction of Bioethics: Cases as Literary Texts* (New York: Routledge, 1999).

CHAPTER 8

PLOT: FRAMING CONTINGENCY
AND CHOICE IN BIOETHICS
TOD CHAMBERS AND KATHRYN MONTGOMERY

T he term *narrative ethics* is variously understood. It may refer to Aesopian stories that end with a take-home moral or to the vicarious experience provided by reading, especially novel-reading, that educates and exercises moral perception. The tradition stretches from Horace,[1] who early in the first millennium wrote that literature should at once teach and delight, to Wayne Booth[2] and Martha Nussbaum,[3] contemporary scholars who have restored the consideration of literature's moral force to critical and theoretical respectability. Adam Zachary Newton has argued that narrative *is* ethics,[4] and an understanding of plot supports him.

Choice is essential to moral life, but both our options and our predispositions have been conditioned, even created, by social forces in the historical moment and by the momentum of our earlier acts. Narrative captures this inextricable tangle of necessity and freedom in human life, and plot enacts it in the selection and ordering of events and in the quasi-causal implications of its telling. Plot links the complicated and uncertain conditions that may—or may not—be essential ingredients in the events being represented, and then plot traces those conditions over time. The suspense of discovering what has happened and how it all turns out may be part of a plot's effect, but, at the story's close, contingency continues to seem inevitable—at least for these people in this one predicament at this time and place. That the story might have been otherwise lures us to listen to and tell other stories, even to retell this story another day.

Literary theory is concerned with the complexities of such narrative representation. Theorists, particularly the Russian formalists, distinguish story (*fabula*) from plot (*sjuzet*).[5] Story is the actual set of events, while plot is the teller's particular arrangement of those events. Suppose a colleague approaches you and says, "We have a patient who came for a prostatectomy, and as he was getting prepped, the nurses noticed that he wouldn't talk about his family. Really odd. Then, after the surgery, he tells us that his wife and children—even his secretary—all think he's away on a business trip, and he doesn't want us to contact them. Now Mr. Kaufman's bleeding, and we just took him back to the OR...." The story of this narrative could be said to be the plain sequence of events: (1) a man learns he needs surgery, (2) he tells his family he is away on a business trip, (3) after the surgery he tells the health care professionals about the deception, (4) he suffers a complication of surgery.

The plot of your colleague's story, however, is quite different, for it begins with the surgery, adds the nurses' observation as a clue, and then reveals the man's secret: he has undergone a surgical procedure absolutely alone, without the advice and support of those closest to him. What's more, the patient has reaffirmed this wish for an unusual, perhaps unhealthy degree of confidentiality, and now with the additional complication of his return to the OR, your colleague is troubled by it. This version begins in medias res, as Horace said all good narratives do, and highlights the surprising but—it is still hoped—nondetrimental deception of a family and a health care team. By plotting the narrative in this way, your colleague tells a story about his own discomfort and its cause. His story has a different impact from one plotted to begin with the patient's decision to deceive his family or another that opens with his cheerful but rather shaky return home. The plot of your colleague's narrative is not the plot of the patient's story nor of his wife's, each of which would require different information, different endings. Plot thus shapes the meaning of narrative and its effect on its audience.

The first duty of an ethicist or an ethics committee is to understand what has happened in the situation under consideration, to answer the question "What is going on here?"[6] What is—and what is not—the case? In bioethics, as in other case-based endeavors (like legal fact-finding, medical diagnosis, and criminal detection), understanding and interpreting involve the construction of a retrospective account of the events in question. Those events—the apparent facts, the inconsistent details, the participants' divergent views—must all be reconciled in a plausible, if often necessarily hypothetical, plot.

This is not always a simple task. Versions may conflict; the parties may invoke different values; individual interpreters may allege the importance of details that others discount or ignore. The process of making sense of a case is inseparable from the interpreter's perception of the values that the case represents. Yet, as if to redeem this subjectivity, the case can be reviewed and reinterpreted. This openness to revision is not a sign of meaninglessness or of relativism but is the condition of our knowledge in the human sciences. In moral matters, as in historiography, narrative is central to *how* we know. Far from yielding to relativism, the recognition of the narrative epistemology of bioethical knowing enables us to represent that knowledge honestly.

PLOT AND NARRATIVE KNOWLEDGE

There are no unplotted stories. Every narrator shapes the story to tell the tale. The selection and ordering of events present each singular narrator's particular view of the matter; every plot is a bid to establish a vision of the truth. Even the attempt to abstract the bare facts into a general, purely chronological outline produces a rudimentary plot.[7] Thus, despite our intuition, there is no "story" without a "plot." The presentation above of the "plain sequence of events" in Mr. Kaufman's case is still a plot, simply one that privileges a narrative perspective close to the patient's point of view. This does not mean, however, that the patient would tell the narrative in this way, for he might begin by relating how he first suspected he was ill and then continue with memories of how his wife became distraught when he was in the hospital ten years ago. Thus one cannot separate plot from point of view. How would his wife tell the story? Or his business partner? Or a client who has been thinking about taking her business elsewhere? How would the surgeon's other colleagues tell it? These are the questions your colleague has begun to ask, questions that ethicists must try to answer.

The knowledge that narrative offers is always situated in the time and place and person of its telling. Plot is not only narrator-dependent; it is performance-dependent, too, contingent upon the relation between a particular teller and par-ticular listeners. The folklorist Richard Bauman observes that when stories are told, they raise not only the question "What is going on *there*?" but a parallel (and related) one: "What is going on *here*?"[8] "Here" to Bauman is the ongoing social sit-uation of the people at the scene of the actual storytelling, and it is part of human nature to try to interpret their actions. "There" refers to the narrative itself and the actions of the imagined actors in the story. Not only does the teller shape the story, but the teller's plot is constructed so that what is going on in the narrative affects what is going on *here* where the story is being told. During the storytelling event, we relate the imagined action (happening *there*) to the ongoing actions of our pre-sent situation (happening *here*), drawing moral, psychological, and sometimes political conclusions. Stories do not exist in an abstract platonic realm but are always embedded in the social interaction of their telling. Ross Chambers reminds us that to study narrative without attending to the "point" of telling that story is to miss the crucial element that conditions the way stories are told; in other words, we are always performing social actions with stories.[9] The context thus does not merely play a role in the act of interpretation but rather is constitutive of the tale's meaning. Consider Mr. Kaufman's story told by his surgeon in the following con-texts. The surgeon relates it to a formal meeting of the ethics committee while Mr. Kaufman is still in the hospital. A month later the surgeon tells a colleague over a casual dinner. A few years later the surgeon relates it to a troubled senior resident during a discussion of a similar situation. In each situation, the story is part of a very different social event: the deliberation by others about one's own actions, a sharing of an interesting experience, or a moment of teaching and counseling. In each situation, the surgeon will replot the story to respond to and to influence social events.

Every presentation of an ethics case therefore needs to be understood as a storytelling event. For this reason, ethicists or ethics committees hear from several perspectives, taking into account the variant plots and the differing goals of sur-geon, nurse, hospital lawyer, and ethicist. However objective each teller's effort, he or she, in the very act of telling, is persuading listeners to take a particular position by shaping the telling of the events in a particular way. This emplotment of the story permits the narrator to make or imply causal connections and thus to lead the listener to understand the narrative the way the teller does.

When an ethics consultation is called, the committee that assembles banks on a history (itself inevitably narrative) of cases heard and resolved in particular ways, and its members have a history of interaction both in ethics deliberations and, for many of them, in the rest of their work lives. How Mr. Kaufman's case is presented and plotted will influence the committee's deliberation and perhaps determine its outcome. How has the individual ethicist or the committee responded to such cases in the past? And how do the committee members respond to one another when considering cases in general? The scope and authority of professionals are often at stake. Someone on the committee who admires Mr. Kaufman's independence may challenge the habit of regarding the patient simply as someone with a socially prescribed role to play. Plotting Mr. Kaufman's case as a story of deception may elicit quite different responses from plotting it as the intern's or nurse's failure to obtain a good social history. A deception story might lead to a quick decision to call the family since there is now no one to make emergency decisions for Mr. Kaufman. The hospital has been deceived! The surgeon's work made more difficult! The expectation of patient confidentiality abused! A fault-finding plot may mobilize long-standing tensions between surgery and nursing or between clinicians and administrators or lead to a recommendation for new hospital rules. If the admirer of independence on the committee is to be persuasive, she will replot the deception—however hypothetically—as the solution to a crisis in Mr. Kaufman's life, a crisis that could be worsened by contacting his family.

Thus, plot should always be seen as a rhetorical construct, for it entails an attempt to portray a particular view of events and their causal antecedents and an effort to shape the consequences. There is always a need to represent the story that the patient could have told and, in Mr. Kaufman's case, a need to imagine his family's account as well. Although the raw materials may seem to be the same, different tellings result in different plots that may lead to very different endings. The nurse or physician who plots Mr. Kaufman's case in a way that culminates in the dramatic revelation of his potentially dangerous decision to keep his surgery secret poses a very different problem from a telling that plots his secrecy as an effort merely to keep personally embarrassing information away from others. Imagine the story being told by Mr. Kaufman to the surgeon. In such a storytelling situation, the patient tells the narrative in order to persuade the surgeon to keep his hospital stay a secret. Or imagine the story being told by the surgeon to the ethics committee; in this situation, the surgeon does not simply present the "facts" but also attempts to persuade the ethics committee of the importance of telling Mr. Kaufman's family by dramatically revealing the secret after telling about the sudden medical complication. And if the story is told by a hospital administrator to a lawyer, the administrator will probably foreground the relation of this narrative to legal problems the hospital has had to face concerning confidentiality.

Plot *is* meaning. Plot shapes a story to represent the significance of its events and to reveal their meaning for the teller and (the teller hopes) the listeners. This ultimate meaning informs the plot, determining the selection and presentation of events. If the word *plot* is used to suggest shaping power in such fields as land surveying and artistic design, it surely suggests how literary plot shapes our narrative perception of experience as "events."[10]

Every story can be retold, replotted, and reinterpreted. New events may be discovered or discerned, and old ones may be given a new causal and temporal construction. Far from being a disadvantage, such recasting is essential to turning medical events into ethics cases. The plot of the conventional medical narrative focuses almost exclusively on details technically salient to medical care. Who the patient is, what she does for a living, her family, her values, and her life goals make little difference in the medical case. It is concerned with the bodily malfunction for which the patient has sought help. Everything personal is secondary to the physical entry of the patient into the clinical spotlight and the clinical investigation that follows: "This the first General Hospital admission for Mr. Kaufman, a forty-three-year-old man who presented to his primary care physician a month ago complaining of…." When Mr. Kaufman's malady is diagnosed, the case will be all but closed: only the denouement of successful therapy customarily follows. If there is an unexpected complication, that's another story, another case. Ideally, nothing will distinguish this case from any other instance of the same malady or any other occurrence of a not uncommon complication of surgery. This loss of individuality is part of the admirable, but sometimes appalling, egalitarian character of medicine. A bioethics case, by contrast, reintroduces character and motivation and thus thickens the plot.

CASES AS TEMPORALLY PLOTTED

It is easy to forget during an ethics consultation that cases are stories and thus are rhetorically plotted. When considering a case, it is instructive to ask how its plot ("what is going on there") is influencing the decisions being made ("what is going on here"). Much can be learned by replotting a story from the perspective of other participants. This is at once an exercise in empathy, a way of revealing the rhetorical stance of the preliminary account, and a means of widening perspective in search of a durable understanding of the case.

Plot can be a matter of life and death. Warren Reich illustrates this in "The Case of the White Oaks Boy," his article on perinatal and neonatal ethics.[11] Written in the first person, the case begins with the narrator, an ethicist, waiting in a conference room at a developmental facility for the arrival of the other members of an ethics committee. A resident arrives and tells him about "Michael," a twenty-one-year-old with a mental age of a two-year-old. The young physician's account begins as a conventional medical case presentation and then deviates from the pattern (as ethics cases often do[12]) to describe the questions Michael's caretakers have about his quality of life. Finally, the ethicist goes with the resident to meet Michael, a meeting that conveys the ethicist's sense of a life without a time frame, one lived in something like an eternal present. Reich plots the case as three accounts folded into one: the ethicist-narrator's, the physician's, and, more indirectly, Michael's. Through the various narrators of this story, the reader vicariously experiences the case as the ethicist's consultative event, as the physician's clinical problem, and finally as Michael's plotless and timeless world. In Reich's story, the reader moves from the outside world and its view of profound mental impairment toward an epiphanic glimpse into Michael's reality. The movement of the plot from impartial outsider to an empathic caretaker to Michael himself leads us to see his life in many ways and to experience the weight of making decisions about him.

The power of storytelling is thus not trivial, and emplotment is central to its capacity for defining issues, describing roles, and determining action. Storytellers cannot evade this authority, and the fact that some parties to a controversy may be silenced implicitly recognizes this. Ethicists may face a bewildering profusion of plots and must choose among them and defend the grounds of their choice.

Two precautions seem advisable. First, ethics cases that seem to have simple plots—Mr. Kaufman as an obvious case of patient autonomy, for example, or as an outrageous instance of patient insubordination—deserve further investigation. An imaginative trial of reemplotment will reveal ethical themes and positions that at first are unrepresented. For example, in a theater exercise, Bertolt Brecht is said to have asked actors to retell the folktale "Goldilocks and the Three Bears" from the perspective of one of the chairs. This shift in point of view engenders a radically different plot: a violent break-in by a malevolent intruder. Such replotting of unduly simple plots can signal underlying yet silent complications, complications perhaps repressed by the story's context. The plot of Mr. Kaufman's own story would probably have begun many years ago, perhaps even in his childhood, although such remote autobiographical plot elements might not be seen as relevant in the context of the hospital.

Second, unlike cases with simple plots, cases with too many possible plots require judicious pruning. The fact that every plot must exclude some considerations as irrelevant behooves ethicists to consider the power calculations that govern storytelling; it does not require ethicists to include everything. How relevant is the surgeon's outrage at Mr. Kaufman's refusal to have his family called? It will depend on the ethical justification it receives (patients have duties too), or the surgeon's institutional power (he's being courted by a rival hospital), or the stories that are hypothetical consequences of that refusal (Mr. Kaufman worsens without anyone to consent to further treatment; he dies and his wife sues). The choice of plot is an ethical decision, and so, too, is the negotiation of that decision. Ethical deliberation, as every hospital administrator understands, is an exercise of power, and it takes place where some might least expect it: in decisions about how a story will be told.

THE CASE IS CLOSED

Cases, like all ways of representing the world, need closure. Aesthetic closure, according to Barbara Herrnstein Smith, occurs when a reader or listener has "the expectation of nothing."[13] This is the moment of stasis when readers feel that nothing can be added to a work. Closure in narrative can be considered in two ways: this conclusion of the interpretive process or the literal end of the story.

Interpretive closure is achieved when there are no more questions to be answered—a satisfying wholeness has been achieved in the tellers' and listeners' sense of what has happened. Their reconstruction of events—their narrative replotting—must be at once full enough to account for what has happened and economical enough to exclude irrelevant detail. This closure is not so much structural as it is epistemological. The plot has been tested against all the available information as it has been variously represented. Earlier hypothetical plots have raised questions, prompted hunches, or defied closure in the structural sense; they have been rejected or refined. Interpretive closure is reached when the narrative can account for the anomalies revealed in the course of the investigation, answer questions raised, and make room for new information. With interpretive closure, plot remains revisable. New information or, as in historiography, a future audience may someday reopen the case. This openness to revision is an aspect of the local and situated narrative knowing characteristic of bioethics—as well as law, history, and the human sciences generally—that enables us to represent that knowledge honestly.

Narrative theorists observe that the events of a plot are often driven by the ending, the second type of closure. So important is structural closure that Walter Benjamin has declared that death is what authorizes narrative and makes stories tellable.[14] Frank Kermode finds in all narrative the "sense of an ending"; for him, the human animal brings order to the world by creating endings to life's various plots.[15] Although cultural anthropologists like Renato Rosaldo[16] and feminist literary critics like Anne Cranny-Francis[17] may wish to challenge Kermode's universalizing of this sense of an ending, the expectations readers have of ethics cases are no different from those they have of other narratives in our culture. Consultations arise out of the need to find a solution to a conflict or a puzzle; the need for closure is also a desire to bring order to what seems to be moral disarray. Ethics committees or ethicists enter the ethics narrative relatively late in its unfolding, truly in medias res, and are asked to help write an ending. But they are not the authors. The duty of the ethicist is not so much to end the story—the patient's attending physician or a hospital lawyer could readily do that. It is rather to envision an ending—or more than one—to the unfolding story. The ethics enterprise is both a part of and separate from the ongoing conflict within the hospital, and its mission is to assist others in constructing one or more acceptable endings to the story.

But what is acceptable? Are the committee members guided toward endings that bring social harmony? Or is it the committee's task to envision endings that provide moral closure but may increase social tension? The recommendation in

Mr. Kaufman's case may create a crisis in his family or it may leave clinicians feeling vulnerable and poorly supported. The pleasure that Warren Reich's Michael takes in his doctor's shiny stethoscope weighs in the balance with his severely limited existence. If plots are driven by their endings, then what is considered a proper ending will have a profound impact on the story that is told. The sense of an ending that can bring closure to moral problems is arbitrary, perhaps temporary, and always a human construction. These limitations are not negative features but rather, when fully recognized, the very business of bioethics.

NOTES

1. Horace, *The Art of Poetry*, trans. Burton Raffel (Albany: State University of New York Press, 1974).
2. Wayne Booth, *The Company We Keep: An Ethics of Fiction* (Berkeley: University of California Press, 1988).
3. Martha C. Nussbaum, *Love's Knowledge: Essays on Philosophy and Literature* (New York: Oxford University Press, 1990).
4. Adam Zachary Newton, *Narrative Ethics* (Cambridge, MA: Harvard University Press, 1997).
5. Lee T. Lemon and Marion J. Reis, eds. and trans., *Russian Formalist Criticism* (Lincoln: University of Nebraska Press, 1965).
6 . The sociologist Erving Goffman noted that as individuals attend to a social interaction they encounter this fundamental interpretive question; see Erving Goffman, *Frame Analysis* (Cambridge, MA: Harvard University Press, 1974), 8.
7. Hayden White distinguishes among annals, chronicle, and history in "The Value of Narrativity in the Representation of Reality," in *On Narrative*, ed. W. J. T. Mitchell (Chicago: University of Chicago Press, 1981), 1–23.
8. Richard Bauman, *Story, Performance, and Event* (Cambridge: Cambridge University Press, 1986), 6.
9. Ross Chambers, *Story and Situation: Narrative Seduction and the Power of Fiction* (Minneapolis: University of Minnesota Press, 1984).
10. Peter Brooks, *Reading for the Plot: Design and Intention in Narrative* (Cambridge, MA: Harvard University Press, 1984).
11. Warren T. Reich, "Caring for Life in the First of It: Moral Paradigms for Perinatal and Neonatal Ethics," *Seminars in Perinatology* 11, no. 3 (1987): 279–87.
12. Tod Chambers, "What to Expect from an Ethics Case (and What It Expects from You)," in *Stories and Their Limits: Narrative Approaches to Bioethics*, ed. Hilde Lindemann Nelson (New York: Routledge, 1998), 171–84.
13. Barbara Herrnstein Smith, *Poetic Closure: A Study of How Poems End* (Chicago: University of Chicago Press, 1968), 34.
14. Walter Benjamin, "The Storyteller," in *Illuminations*, ed. Hannah Arendt, trans. Harry Zohn (New York: Schocken Books, 1969), 83–110.
15. Frank Kermode, *The Sense of an Ending: Studies in the Theory of Fiction* (New York: Oxford University Press, 1967).
16. Renato Rosaldo, *Culture and Truth: The Remaking of Social Analysis* (Boston: Beacon Press, 1989).
17. Anne Cranny-Francis, *Feminist Fiction: Feminist Uses of Generic Fiction* (Oxford: Polity Press, 1990).

CHAPTER 9

THE READER'S RESPONSE AND WHY IT MATTERS IN BIOMEDICAL ETHICS
CHARLES M. ANDERSON AND MARTHA MONTELLO

[A] real book reads us. I have been read by Eliot's poems and by Ulysses *and by* Remembrance of Things Past *and by* The Castle *for a good many years now, since early youth. Some of these books at first rejected me; I bored them. But as I grew older and they knew me better, they came to have more sympathy with me and to understand my hidden meanings.*

—*Lionel Trilling, "On the Teaching of Modern Literature"*

When he was first diagnosed with prostate cancer, Anatole Broyard, the well-known literary critic for the *New York Times Book Review*, wrote, "[W]hat I want in a doctor...[is]...one who is a close reader of illness....I want to be a good story for my doctor, to exchange some of my art for his."[1] This highly articulate patient recognized that we comprehend our own and each other's lives through the stories that define us. Constructing time-bound, causal patterns enables us to make sense of primary experience. The narratives we build shape the ways we come to know ourselves and each other and create the symbolic space within which we make all our moral choices.[2] Broyard understood that, with his illness and its attendant physical and emotional suffering and difficult moral decisions, he would need a competent reader as desperately as he would need a competent physician.

Of all the literary elements that come into play when we read or hear a narrative, it is the reader's role that is most often undervalued when we explore the meaning of a story. We readily acknowledge the critical importance of plot, context, voice, time, and character, but what difference does it make who is doing the reading? What happens to us and through us when we read? Why and how do so many different meanings emerge from the same narrative when different readers from different times and places experience it? What consequences might an understanding of reader roles have for the practice of biomedical ethics? We believe the consequences are enormous because it is the reader's role in the narratives of moral deliberation that most directly and powerfully connects the experience of literature with the deliberative processes of biomedical ethics.

The case we want to build for paying attention to the role of the reader in bio-medical ethics is a complicated one. It begins with contemporary literary theory defining the active role of the reader, moves to fifth-century Athens and the beginning of Western ethics in order to discover highly active readers at the very genesis of Western ethical method and intention, and then returns to the world of contemporary medical care, where we hope to demonstrate that understanding the reader's role matters a great deal when difficult moral decisions must be made.

READER-RESPONSE CRITICAL THEORIES

The text-oriented theories dominating early-twentieth-century literary criticism paid scant attention to the reader's role. Meaning in a literary work was to be found "out there," in the words on the page. Unlike earlier traditions espousing more humanistic or integrative approaches to literary texts, the so-called New Critics of the 1940s and 1950s generally insisted on the autonomy of the work itself, which could be interpreted through close, systematic reading and detailed textual analysis.[3] Biography, personality, and intention of the author as well as cultural and historical contexts mattered less than internal consistency, allusion, and the clever resolution of ambiguity. Taking their cue from positivist success in other fields, literary critics of this time made reading more systematic by eliminating the most troublesome element in the literary process, the reader. Confusing "the work" with its psychological and emotional effects, they insisted, constituted an "affective fallacy" that resulted in a distorting relativism and an untrustworthy subjectivism.[4]

Since the mid-1970s, however, serious critical attention has shifted to focus on the reader's experience of reading and has invited discussion about personal engagement, emotions, and values.[5] Scholars have examined the cognitive, emotional, and psychological responses set in motion by words on the page in the reader during the act of reading.[6] The subjectivity of the reader, not the autonomy of the text, is at the center of this critical attention. Meaning is understood to take shape—for different critics in different ways and to different degrees—in the symbolic space that reader, text, and other elements create during the reading process and does not exist without the subjective activity and the contextual elements brought to the text by each reader.[7]

By placing the reader at the center of the symbolic processes from which meaning arises, reader-response critics returned to a very old intellectual movement described in the work of early-twentieth-century philosophers and rhetoricians. The central concerns of this movement are most succinctly expressed in philosopher Ernst Cassirer's *Essay on Man*:

> [M]an lives in a symbolic universe. Language, myth, art, and religion are parts of this universe. They are the varied threads which weave the symbolic net, the tangled web of human experience. All human progress in thought and experience refines upon and

strengthens this net. No longer can man confront reality immediately; he cannot see it, as it were, face to face. Physical reality seems to recede in proportion as man's symbolic activity advances.... He has so enveloped himself in linguistic forms, in artistic images, in mythical symbols or religious rites that he cannot see or know anything except by the interposition of this artificial medium.... He lives... in the midst of imaginary emotions, in hopes and fears, in illusions and disillusions, in his fantasies and dreams. "What disturbs and alarms man," said Epictetus, "are not the things, but his opinions and fancies about the things."[8]

Later in the same essay, Cassirer redefines man not as *animal rationale* but as *animal symbolicum*, not as the rational animal, but as the symbol-using animal (p. 26). If Cassirer and others who make similar arguments are correct, then the meaning-making that happens between the pages of a good book also happens in the moment-to-moment living of all men and women as they work to make sense of experience. For our purposes, it makes the transition from novel, poem, and critical abstraction to the everyday process of significant moral decision-making natural, sensible, and, as we shall see in the next section, essential.

NARRATIVE IN ETHICAL DISCOURSE

Narratives constructed from the stuff of daily life have always been powerful and necessary aspects of Western ethical discourse, whose fundamental processes of moral decision-making and reasoning, we believe, have always been narrative in nature. To support this assertion, we turn to the *Gorgias*, an early and powerful statement of Plato's view of what ethics ought to be about and how ethical discourse and deliberation should be performed.[9] Plato's text will show us exactly how contemporary reader-response theory and ethical deliberation converge in ways that may prove helpful to our understanding and practice of narrative ethics in the medical encounter.

In the dialogue, Socrates meets a group of people making their way home after a demonstration by the famous and respected sophist Gorgias, for whom the dialogue is named. Having missed the demonstration, Socrates begins the conversation by asking Gorgias "what the power of his art consists in and what it is that he professes and teaches" (p. 19). Socrates then engages three different auditors: first Gorgias, then the much younger and less experienced orator Polus, and finally the powerful and dangerous politician Callicles. He asks each to participate in what we know as the Socratic method or dialectic, in which one person asks, the other answers; terms and concepts are divided and divided again, defined and redefined; and the goal is to convince one another and thereby to arrive at "absolute truth" (p. 84). The ethical truth to be examined this particular evening is the unconventional and outrageous assertion that it is better to suffer wrong than to do wrong and its even more outrageous corollary—that the only greater evil is not to be punished for doing wrong.

Much of the dialogue seems narrow and unrelenting, with Socrates appearing to use whatever strategies he can to demolish and destroy his opposition—at least that is what Polus and Callicles accuse him of doing, and that is how many who claim to practice the Socratic method understand it to work. Socrates, however, denies that he is only out to win, volunteers to switch sides, and characterizes his interlocutors as his friends, begging them time and again not to fall back, but to consider his best interests as he considers theirs, to correct him in whatever way he has gone astray. We believe Socrates is sincere when he claims not to be interested in the winning or losing of arguments, but in precisely what he tells us he is interested in: friendship, but friendship of a very particular kind.

The friendship Plato through Socrates espouses here and throughout his dialogues is a friendship dedicated to overcoming the distance between self and other, a friendship that cares more for the friend than for the self.[10] Rooted in what rhetorician Kenneth Burke describes as the natural inclination of persons to "identify" with others, Socrates' greatest form of friendship seeks "consubstantiality," which is the recognition that, despite significant differences, I am of the same substance as you, we share interests, experiences, and we value each other accordingly.[11] Identification and consubstantiality encourage us to let go of ourselves and to trust that we will not be betrayed by those with whom we are friends. Again and again, Socrates tells us that without such a friendship and the honest, loving dialogue it engenders, the philosopher cannot find the wisdom he seeks.

Throughout the *Gorgias*, Socrates uses a variety of narratives to reason with his interlocutors. Again and again, he shifts the conversation to the most common of everyday stories, such as those of shoemakers and athletic training. These shifts serve two crucial functions: (1) they introduce a contrapuntal rhythm, moving the interlocutors and the audience from thought to image, argument to experience, and back again to enrich and deepen the participation necessary to Socrates' particular form of narrative reasoning; and (2) they actualize or, as Aristotle might put it, "bring before the eyes" the concrete material realities suggested by the more or less abstract arguments made throughout the discussion.[12] As his interlocutors imaginatively enter the "virtual" worlds Socrates offers them, they discover that their ethical positions, no matter how compelling, generally accepted, or logically defensible, lead directly to realities that are simply uninhabitable. James Boyd White, in his remarkable book *When Words Lose Their Meaning: Constitutions and Reconstitutions of Language, Character, and Community*, describes and analyzes the scene in which Socrates employs one such narrative to show Callicles that the orderly man is happier than the licentious man:

> Imagine two men, he says, each with a number of jars to be filled with wine, honey, or milk. The jars of one are sound and full, and he wants nothing; the jars of the other are leaky, and he must constantly struggle to keep them full. Does this image not portray the difference between the life of one who wants nothing and the life of one who is constantly scurrying after pleasures? (493e–494a). This fable is not addressed to the intellectual part of Callicles but to the part of his mind that thinks and feels in images. It asks him to imagine what it would really be like . . . to be a leaky jar, constantly run-

ning out and being refilled, and an owner in frantic motion, constantly filling, and what, on the contrary, it would be like to be sound and full and at rest.... The self takes more than one form, here both jar and owner, and the story is about deep feelings within the self: anxiety and loss versus security and gain.[13]

At another point in the *Gorgias*, Socrates demonstrates what he sees as the consequences of Polus's conventional arguments regarding political expediency and rule by the most powerful by offering him a narrative image of Athens's walls breached by enemies, its fleet burning in the harbor. This is a vision Polus, given his sincere desire to serve the state, cannot bring himself to inhabit. If he denounces the narrative Socrates reveals to him, he must also denounce the reasoning that created it, abandon his earlier position, and open himself to the possibility of a more profound engagement in the ethics of Athenian politics. If he refuses to denounce it, he violates the core values by which he lives: love for his city and patriotic service to it. What is at stake here is not the winning of an argument or the completion of an entertaining story but the changing of lives. Should Polus decide in error, Athens may burn.

The ethical wisdom necessary to make the decisions demanded by this and other Platonic dialogues depends upon the willingness of Socrates' interlocutors to engage narrative in exactly the ways reader-response criticism suggests that readers engage all literary texts, in the way Cassirer tells us that we live in the world, in the way Broyard and the physician-reader he sought would engage the story of his illness. Socrates invites us to join him, to imaginatively experience the narrative realities coiled within the arguments set before us, to inhabit those realities as fully as possible, and then to return to the present moment to consider in a more critical, more analytical way the knowledge gleaned from the experience. In this process, the destabilization of self that results when one gives oneself over to the rhetorical power of the narrative is balanced by the stabilizing influence of critical conventions, analytical methodologies, and the relational impact of the friendship shared by the participants in the conversation.[14] Rational and experiential, emotional and logical, this reading process requires that every participant—writer and reader—bring to the experience everything he or she knows and is in order to make as fully informed and ethically inhabitable a decision as possible. We believe that this is precisely what the practice of empathic, compassionate medicine and effective bioethical deliberation require as well.

NARRATIVE REASONING IN BIOETHICAL DELIBERATION

We confess that we are not completely certain how the narrative reasoning and reader roles experienced in the encounters and theories we have been describing can be "applied" to biomedical ethics. Unlike the systematic application of the four principles or the objective grid in the introduction to Jonsen, Siegler, and Winslade's *Clinical Ethics*, our methods are elusive, difficult to quantify or to precisely control.[15] But because these methods are crucial to and already present in moral decision-making, we must consider not simply the potential consequences of new narrative methods in bioethics. More important, we need to examine the effects narrative reasoning already *has* on moral deliberation and on the various parties in the medical encounter. We offer two cases, one a cautionary tale and the other a utopian narrative of how it might be.

Mrs. X is a forty-one-year-old patient with a long history of infertility. She has undergone extensive work-up for this problem, including multiple cycles of in vitro fertilization. Two years ago, in vitro fertilization resulted in a twin pregnancy. However, a complication of her ovarian stimulation led to ovarian hyperstimulation syndrome, for which she was hospitalized for five days and subsequently lost her twin gestation. Now, two years later, she has undergone another cycle of in vitro fertilization, which has produced a quadruplet pregnancy.

She presented at seven weeks in search of an obstetrician who practices high-risk obstetrics. Her initial questions and those of her husband centered on the physician's practice style and the delivery setting. They asked his opinion on the issue of fetal reduction to a twin pregnancy to improve outcome.

The couple later broached the subject of genetic mapping of the quadruplet pregnancy. This entails chorionic villi sampling of all the placental beds of the four fetuses at roughly nine to eleven weeks, before amniocentesis can be performed, in order to determine their genetic makeup. Since she was forty-one years old, accumulative risk for Down's syndrome in one of the infants was almost one in four. The physician referred the couple to an out-of-state hospital for this procedure, which was performed on all four fetuses.

In the interim between the procedure, the reception of its results, and the use of those results to make the decision to reduce to two fetuses, the couple asked the physician's advice regarding sex selection. They hoped to reduce to a male and a female fetus. The couple chose to reduce to a male-female twin pregnancy, which was carried to term. She delivered two live infants by elective cesarean, and is now learning to be a parent of twins.

This case is clearly a very complex narrative with at least as much omitted as has been included. It was originally presented by the physician involved to an ethics class at a major American medical school. When small groups of students were asked to consider the ethical dimensions of the case, confusion descended upon the group. They needed more information: How dangerous was the test? What is the usual procedure in such a case? Did selecting the two fetuses by sex endanger the gestation and delivery process? At some point in one of the groups, a student, frustrated by the complexity and ambiguity of the case, blurted out something like: "Next thing you know, they'll want a blond-haired, blue-eyed yuppie with a date book attached!"

After a moment's silence, the room exploded into discussion. Once the students had a moral characterization of the participants in this narrative, they also had a story line that allowed them to express both their thoughts and feelings and their frustration over the case. The interesting, cautionary aspect is that they had an extremely difficult time returning to a more objective or balanced reading of the story. They understood that the comment had unfairly transformed the couple into perpetuators of Nazi eugenics experimentation, but their entry into that story line made it hard for them to imagine the couple as two deeply loving human beings, willing to devote everything in their lives to caring for the children they hoped to bring into the world, an equally plausible characterization that would move narrative, reader, and the interpretive community into a significantly different relationship with the case and with the people involved in it.

One response to the narrative issuing from this case might be to call for more emphasis on objectivity, not less. However, our experience and a considerable body of work in narrative ethics and related areas tell us that stark mathematical or logical objectivity is simply not possible in the world of human interactions.[16] This being so, attending to the desires, emotions, and moral understandings the students brought to their attempt to construct a meaningful, ethically inhabitable encounter with the couple above becomes crucially important. We cannot imagine that the quality of care for the couple above would not be negatively influenced by the narrative the students used to define them and to understand their interests. Another response might be that the students lack the sophistication of practitioners, but the kind of reasoning we see in this case is not limited to inexperienced students. We can all remember instances in which unexamined narrative reasoning has produced devastatingly unethical consequences: the Tuskegee syphilis experiments, responses to the early AIDS epidemic, the case of Dax Cowart. Whether we want to or not, we bring everything we are to moral encounters, and everything we bring shapes how we as readers and co-composers of moral narratives act, for good or ill. While there is great danger in such open, active participation, there is also great opportunity. Our second "case" addresses this opportunity.

In "'Forty Acres of Cotton Waiting to Be Picked': Medical Students, Storytelling, and the Rhetoric of Healing," I (Anderson) explore the impact of narratives upon the formation of the physician.[17] Near the end of the article, I introduce the story of Mrs. Green, "a train wreck" who has been admitted to the hospital for numerous complaints of end-stage diabetes. The harried medical student who attempts to take her history is appalled by the "case" before him, until he accidentally opens a door onto the narrative of the patient's life by casually remarking that "she had undoubtedly seen a lot of cotton being raised in her lifetime" (p. 292). The symbolic invitation offered by the student's comment produces remarkable results:

> The moans were immediately stifled. I . . . watched her expression change as her mind took her back to a time and place she had not visited in a very long while. Her facial expression softened, her breathing patterns became quieter, her limbs became still. After several moments, she began to speak. She did not speak in the halting, grammatically impoverished style that had plagued me during my history and physical, but spoke in a flowing manner that is so characteristic of Southerners.

Mrs. Green spoke of cotton-chopping, the method of hoeing weeds out of cotton fields commonly practiced before the onslaught of herbicides and modern cultivating machinery. She talked of the long rides in the back of a truck to the fields, the dust that rose with your hoe as you made your way...with dozens of other choppers. How sweet the water tasted when you finally made it down the long row and back. She described how the grasshoppers would greet them with a song upon their arrival, and how these same grasshoppers would bid them farewell at the end of the day. Sack lunches of fried chicken, cornbread, and a Moon-Pie for dessert. Two dollars for a hard day's labor. Oh, and the blisters, those terrible, God-awful blisters. (P. 293)

Over the course of his treatment of Mrs. Green, the student, who grew up on a farm in the same area of the Arkansas Delta, finds himself transformed by the narrative consubstantiality they share. As he resists and finally discards the normative medical narrative of the "train wreck" and opens himself to other possibilities, the medical student comes to know that what has been derailed is not Mrs. Green's body, but the story that gives meaning to the events that body has experienced over its lifetime. As he enters the world her story offers him, he meets her authentic, historic self and understands that she and he, as different as they might seem, are indeed of the same substance at the deepest levels of human experience and value. He is empowered by that knowledge to deliver effective, efficient medical care that brings about significant improvement in her physical, psychological, and social conditions, medical care he simply could not deliver had he not so fully participated in the narrative events in which her story engages him. In the end, Mrs. Green's narrative transformation from "train wreck" to teacher to mother to loving friend alters and enriches the student as profoundly as it enriches her and the ones she has loved, lost, and found again:

She had made contact with her family again, not the family she had known in the nursing home, but the family that she had raised, cared for, and labored for. And unbeknownst to her, she had made contact with a rather naïve medical student and had introduced him to the simple healing power of a hand offered in kindness. (Pp. 296–97)

As Anatole Broyard recognized the centrality of story to his condition, so do we recognize the centrality of narrative to this case both to its telling and to its subsequent effective treatment. Surely something like the narrative repair that takes place for Mrs. Green and her physician and what Broyard longed for in the interchange with his doctor is what Socrates had in mind for all of Athenian society when he invited his friends to join him in his search for the truth so long ago in the home of Callicles, and it is certainly what we have in mind when we argue that serious attention to the reader's role in the narrative reasoning of biomedical ethics matters a great deal.

At the end of the *Gorgias*, Socrates appears to have won all the arguments and to have humiliated and demolished his foes, but in fact he and all of Athens have lost. Because his interlocutors could not move beyond the constraints of their own argumentative positions, because they could not overcome the distance between self and other and bring themselves to take the risks associated with the quality of friendship he offered them, Socrates, unlike Mrs. Green, Anatole Broyard, and their physicians, stands alone, exposed, without friends, without a shared understanding of how a good life might be lived in this place at this time under these hard conditions. The greatest danger in Socrates' world (and in our own) lies in the failure of individuals to engage in the dialogue between reader and text or between the self and other, to immerse themselves in the stories that surround them, for it is in the dialogue, and there alone, that we experience the rhythms of asking and answering, speaking and listening, feeling and thinking, giving and receiving that lie at the center of the work we do, not the *either/or* but the *and/also* of compassionate moral deliberation and ethical decision-making.

NOTES

1. Anatole Broyard, "Doctor, Talk to Me," in *New York Times Magazine* (August 26, 1990), 35–36.
2. Jerome Bruner, *Actual Minds, Possible Worlds* (Cambridge, MA: Harvard University Press, 1986); Margaret Urban Walker, *Moral Understandings: A Feminist Study in Ethics* (New York: Routledge, 1998); and Alisdair McIntyre, *After Virtue* (Notre Dame, IN: Notre Dame University Press, 1981).
3. One of the most influential critical studies of the time was Austin Warren and René Wellek, *Theory of Literature* (New York: Harcourt, Brace, 1949).
4. W. K. Wimsatt and Monroe Beardsley, "The Affective Fallacy," in W. K. Wimsatt, *The Verbal Icon: Studies in the Meaning of Poetry* (Lexington: University Press of Kentucky, 1949).
5. Wayne Booth, *The Company We Keep: An Ethics of Fiction* (Berkeley: University of California Press, 1988); Edward Hirsch, *Responsive Reading* (Ann Arbor: University of Michigan Press, 1999); J. A. Appleyard, *Becoming a Reader: The Experience of Fiction from Childhood to Adulthood* (New York: Cambridge University Press, 1990); and Martha Nussbaum, *Love's Knowledge: Essays on Philosophy and Literature* (New York: Oxford University Press, 1990).
6. Richard Gerrig, *Experiencing Narrative Worlds: On the Psychological Activities of Reading* (New Haven: Yale University Press, 1993); and Mark Johnson, *Moral Imagination: Implications of Cognitive Science for Ethics* (Chicago: University of Chicago Press, 1993).
7. Stanley Fish, *Is There a Text in This Class? The Authority of Interpretive Communities* (Cambridge, MA: Harvard University Press, 1980); Norman Holland, "Unity-Identity-Text-Self," *Publications of the Modern Language Association* 90 (October 1975): 812–22; and Wolfgang Iser, *The Act of Reading* (Baltimore: Johns Hopkins University Press, 1978).
8. Ernst Cassirer, *An Essay on Man: An Introduction to a Philosophy of Human Culture* (New Haven: Yale University Press, 1945), 25. Subsequent page references to this work appear in parentheses in the text.
9. In a commentary in *American Journal of Bioethics* 1, no. 1 (Winter 2001): 61–62, Anderson draws on this text to examine related ways that ethical discourse mirrors the

process of deliberation in bioethics. Plato, *Gorgias*, trans. Walter Hamilton (New York: Penguin Classics, 1985). Subsequent page references to this work appear in parentheses in the text.

10. See Plato's much later dialogue *Phaedrus* for a full development of this kind of friendship.

11. Kenneth Burke, *A Rhetoric of Motives* (Berkeley: University of California Press, 1969).

12. Aristotle, *The Rhetoric*, 3.10.

13. James Boyd White, *When Words Lose Their Meaning: Constitutions and Reconstitutions of Language, Character, and Community* (Chicago: University of Chicago Press, 1984), 106. We are deeply indebted to and fully acknowledge White's book for our understanding of Socrates' method in the *Gorgias*. Without his insights, this essay could not have been written.

14. See the first and second speeches in the *Phaedrus* for a description of how the self can be brutalized and lost to narratives experienced outside the friendship Platonic method requires.

15. Albert Jonsen, Mark Siegler, William Winslade, *Clinical Ethics*, 4th ed. (New York: McGraw-Hill, 1982).

16. For example, see Tod Chambers, *The Fiction of Bioethics: Cases as Literary Texts* (New York: Routledge, 1999).

17. Charles Anderson, "'Forty Acres of Cotton Waiting to Be Picked': Medical Students, Storytelling, and the Rhetoric of Healing," *Literature and Medicine* 17 (2000): 280–97.

PART III

CASE STUDIES IN NARRATIVE ETHICS

CHAPTER 10

THE NARRATIVE OF RESCUE IN PEDIATRIC PRACTICE
WALTER M. ROBINSON

The death of a child challenges the order of the world, for it is always premature. We cannot invoke a tale of a long, well-lived life when a child dies, and so we create new stories about innocent suffering, the injustice of the world, the need for heroic rescue, or the pain of tragedy. These stories are the narratives we use to guide our way through the events of life and death: they set the stage for our actions and provide the framework for our beliefs and intentions. In this chapter I will examine how heroic rescue, a common narrative of childhood illness, frames the thinking of pediatricians and parents who are faced with the potential death of a child.[1]

THE NARRATIVE FORM OF PEDIATRICS: NARRATIVES AS CLINICAL TOOLS

Narrative techniques operate in clinical practice as a set of clinical tools. Pediatricians ask questions and listen to a story ("Tell me what brings you to see me today?" "Well, Bobby was doing just fine until last Thursday, when he came home from school with a cough and...") and then organize that information into a stylized, linear narrative, the "presenting history," which can function as a diagnostic and prognostic tool.[2] Gaps in the story elicit more questions ("Was anyone else at school sick?") until bit by bit the patient's story is revealed and translated into the style, content, and language of a medical history.[3]

Pediatrics is more explicitly concerned with families than are most other branches of medicine, and narrative techniques reinforce our understanding of patients not as localized collections of signs and symptoms but as characters in a family story that began before the clinic and will continue after the exam room. As adults, we might all like to view ourselves as the authors of our own story, but working daily with children reminds us of the generational process that produced us and in which we all play a part. Young pediatricians are taught to see the child as one character in the social, emotional, economic, and moral story of the family. This commitment to the family is made explicit by saying, "In pediatrics, the family is the patient."

THE NARRATIVE CONTENT OF PEDIATRICS: THE NARRATIVE OF RESCUE

An important, and perhaps defining, model for the professional practice of pediatrics is the narrative of rescue. This narrative is an organizing set of beliefs and explanations about the work of pediatricians, born both of a contemporary faith in technological progress and of a belief that serious childhood illness is in some deep sense *unnatural*, or outside the expected order of things. That such a narrative can take hold in pediatric practice is a testament to the successes of contemporary medicine; in the prior ages of largely ineffective therapeutics, such a view of childhood illness would have seemed delusional.

The rescue narrative sets up the pediatrician as the rescuer, a heroic warrior against illness and despair. The need to be seen as heroic may be necessary to permit pediatricians to harm children in the pursuit of healing them. While an adult may make sense of the suffering often required to cure a serious illness, a child cannot. Adopting the role of rescuer shields us from both the child's indignation and our own sense that we are harming those whom we intend to protect. We may need this compelling heroic role to allow us to inflict suffering on protesting children, to permit us to make them sicker now so that they may be well later. Yet the rescue narrative also constrains pediatricians by limiting their range of responses to illness and making it particularly difficult to treat a child when a cure—a rescue—is impossible.

NARRATIVES IN MORAL REASONING

Narratives in pediatrics do not supplant ethical principles but precede their invocation and inform their application. Narratives are the substrates for moral reasoning. Faced with ethical issues, pediatricians use narratives to frame the alternatives, explore the options, consider the consequences, and deliberate about right and wrong. Narratives help us see what is at stake in any particular case, outline the nature and scope of any disagreements, and determine the possible options.

The narrative structure of moral reasoning is more apparent in pediatrics because we cannot fall back on notions of individual autonomy to help us out of ethically problematic situations; we cannot take easy refuge in the "out" of letting the patient decide, for the child patient can almost never decide by himself. Because children generally cannot tell us directly about their values, their experiences are more open to interpretation by others than is the case with adults. True, pediatricians are skilled translators of children's behavior into sets of medical signs and symptoms, but on a deeper level, the profession of pediatrics has an internal set of normative assumptions about the best interests of children and about what sort of life is worth living. These normative assumptions frame the boundaries of competent pediatric practice. A narrative of rescue often lies at the center of this framework.

THE NARRATIVES OF FAMILY LIFE

Families also invoke narratives as a way of describing themselves and their goals. Family narratives have characters, some living, some dead; families have stories that persist over generations; families tell internal tales that explicitly or implicitly frame the meaning of the present with the events of the past and the future. Many families see themselves as continuations: they see the smile of Aunt Sally in young Susan or say the baby has Grandpa's green eyes.[4] Family narratives are often the principal means of shaping and describing what counts as a good parent, a good child, and a good life.

Just as we ought not to take the narrative of rescue in pediatric practice at face value, we ought not treat these family narratives as superficial stories of "how life goes in our family." Family stories are messy and may be internally contradictory as well as self-serving. Family stories structure the conflicting events that occur in life and provide a template for teasing out meaning from the confusion of experience. A child plays an especially powerful role in the story of a family, often enacting a plot or playing a role that may have long preceded him or her.

When illness threatens the integrity of the family, the roles children and parents play in the family narrative deserve special attention. In particular, families can be open to the possibility and presence of tragedy, an idea almost completely alien to modern pediatrics. The acceptance of tragedy is disruptive when seen from the high-technology world of pediatrics and can lead parents into direct conflict with physicians and ethics consultants. Families can have a strong sense of the natural and the unnatural and a potent sense of fate and of faith. For some families, the dominant rescue narrative of pediatric practice fits within their own stories of "doing everything." For others, rescue and heroism are irrelevant and even counterproductive to their understanding of the serious illness or death of a child as a tragic event.

NARRATIVES AND ETHICAL CONFLICT

It might seem easier to avoid the messy conflict of professional and family narratives by applying a straightforward principlist method to the ethical issues in pediatrics. We might like to reason that since children do not have autonomy, we need simply to find the appropriate decision-maker for the child—a sort of ethical regent until the child can assume the mantle of his own responsibility—and leave it at that.

The real world intrudes upon these plans. Pediatricians and parents often have vastly different goals for how a child's life or death should go, not to mention different ideas about whether a life is worth living. For pediatricians, defining ethics as simply a set of procedures for determining an appropriate surrogate will seem like a legalistic abdication, since pediatricians have their own narrative of the value and appropriate use of medical care, one that they are unwilling to surrender to any surrogate, no matter how legitimate.

What follows is a discussion of two types of cases in which the dominant rescue narrative of pediatrics conflicts with family narratives. In the first type of case, the rescue narrative starkly contrasts with the family's sense of tragedy and fate. In the second set of cases, the rescue narrative is so dominant that it suppresses the development and expression of any other way of thinking about serious illness and death.

A CASE OF "COGNITIVE SPARING"

When Mark was born, his mother knew that something was terribly wrong. Because he did not begin to breathe, CPR was started in the delivery room. He was quickly placed on a ventilator and developed seizures requiring repeated doses of medication. He was transported to the neonatal intensive care unit of a tertiary pediatric hospital in another state.

An ethics committee report picks up the story ten days later: "Based on serial clinical examinations, brain imaging with MRI, EEG findings, and daily consultation by a pediatric neuro-intensivist, [Mark] is described as having evidence of a significant neurologic injury."

Mark's parents were devastated by the diagnosis and, after some discussion with the clinical team, asked that the ventilator be withdrawn from their son so that he could die, as they put it, "without unnatural delays." When the clinical team expressed some reservations over granting this request, Mark's parents asked for an ethics committee consult. After discussion with the parents, the clinical and ethics committee teams agreed that it was reasonable to remove the ventilator; if the extent of his brain injury were so severe that Mark could not breathe on his own, then the ventilator would not be replaced, and Mark would be "allowed to die."[5]

The ventilator was removed, and, to the surprise of the clinicians and the parents, Mark breathed spontaneously. But he had no suck reflex and no ability to swallow; he did not respond when given a bottle. The clinical team now wanted to place a feeding tube through Mark's nose into his stomach so that formula could be dripped slowly into his stomach. His parents objected, saying that the feeding tube was just another artificial way of keeping Mark alive: Wasn't the feeding tube just like the ventilator, they asked, a way of prolonging Mark's death? In contrast, the clinical team believed that Mark had an unusual brain injury; the consultants used the phrase "cognitive sparing" to describe Mark's future, one that held relatively little mental retardation but included blindness, deafness, and an inability to walk, talk, or even move easily.

In a subsequent letter to the attending physicians, nurses, and ethics committee members, Mark's parents begin with these lines:

> We are asking for your help in arranging palliative care for Mark and advising us regarding options for keeping him comfortable so that he may pass away peacefully and without unnatural delays.... We have searched our hearts and minds from every

angle we could find, and we've constantly prayed for God to guide us in making a decision in Mark's best interest. We have asked questions and listened carefully to all of you for three weeks. We have involved the ethics people and we have listened to opinions and comments from everyone involved.

The letter closes with the paragraph:

We are Mark's parents—Mommy and Daddy. No person on earth loves or wants him so much as we do. But we are willing to let him go to God. And so, we ask you to support us and help us make Mark's passing as comfortable, peaceful, and natural as possible. If and when all artificial measures are removed, we all will truly have turned the decision over to God.

The ethics consultation team also assessed Mark's situation in a report to the parents and the full ethics committee:

Many committee members firmly support the parents' right to make a decision to withdraw all life sustaining treatments. That view is based on the belief that his parents are clearly trying to determine what is best for Mark, and there is sufficient medical uncertainty to defer to the parents as the most ethically appropriate surrogate decision makers for Mark.... On the other hand, many members felt strongly that an irrevocable decision to let Mark die, when it is not known whether he might develop significant cognitive and relational ability, is premature. [Waiting] will enable his parents to weigh more accurately what is best for him and have the long term solace that comes from knowing that a decision was not made until more prognostically useful information was obtained. In addition, given the current ambiguity of his prognosis, concern for protecting infant's rights would suggest that it is prudent to allow time to determine his developmental capacity with more certainty.

The report continues:

While both [the parents and the physicians] agreed that the neurological prognosis cannot be known for certain at this juncture, there were some significant differences on how the information available at this time is interpreted. Mark's parents emphasized concerns that placed the long term quality of life and relational ability at the severe end of the spectrum of possible outcomes outlined by the clinical team.... [The clinical team] expressed concern that it is still too early in the course for a newborn infant having suffered this type of injury and that additional recovery of neurologic function may yet manifest itself.

Let us lay out the differing views of the family and the physicians. Mark's parents interpreted his situation as a living hell, trapped inside a body that could never "work" and tormented by the *awareness of what he was missing*. They viewed this state as made possible only by medical intrusion into what otherwise would have been the peaceful but tragic early death of a child. They feared the greater tragedy of continued life and their helplessness to halt what they saw as the artificial prolongation of tragedy if further delay were permitted.

On the other hand, the clinicians and some members of the ethics team told a story of an exceptional child and used analogies to Christopher Reeve and Helen

Keller in characterizing the possible futures for Mark. They believed that Mark's brain injury was rare ("on the good end of the spectrum"), that he was unlike many other infants they had diagnosed with severe brain injuries, and that his life, while difficult, could be worth living. They were uncertain in this prognosis, and they favored waiting, with more examinations and possibly more brain scans. They felt that if they were wrong, the feeding tube could always be withdrawn later, so that there was no disadvantage in waiting for more information.[6]

At stake here are two different narratives of a life after a severe brain injury at birth, two different stories about how Mark's life will go. The parents tell a story of a tragic accident of fate, a life not meant to be, a life in God's hands. The doctors tell a story of triumph over disability, of possible rescue from tragic fate, of uncertainty requiring more testing and observation. Given these conflicting narratives, it is unavoidable that the possibilities of moral action, "the *morals* of the story," will conflict.

While viewing the difficulties in this case as conflicts between competing narratives does not resolve them, we cannot understand what is at stake in the decision to remove the feeding tube unless we understand the symbolic importance of such an action from within the conflicting narratives. To ignore the narrative context on either side is to reduce the issue to the question "Is it permissible to remove a feeding tube from an infant with a severe brain injury?"—a question that has only a parsimonious and theoretical answer. Any answer that fails to address the conflict in the narratives will also fail to account for the deeply held values on both sides. It will satisfy no one. The common desire to invoke an adult framework for ethical decisions by translating this issue into a question of who decides also misses the point, since both sides have clear and conflicting views of what constitutes Mark's best interest, and neither would be satisfied with the decision made by the other.

Perhaps because of the overwhelming power of the clinical team, in combination with the natural reluctance of the parents to desire, and, further, to *advocate for* the death of their child, the decision was made to institute tube feedings. Mark did not recover any ability to suck or swallow, nor has he yet shown any signs of recovery from his brain injury. Because his family could not manage his medical care at home, he now resides in a nursing home. He is still fed by tube every day.

THE SEDUCTION OF RESCUE: PROGRESS, TECHNOLOGY AND CYSTIC FIBROSIS

The next pair of cases explores the difficulties that occur when the dominant rescue narrative overwhelms the other narratives of pediatric practice; both are drawn from the experience of patients and physicians in a cystic fibrosis clinic.

Cystic fibrosis (CF) is the most common inherited and lethal illness among Caucasians in North America. One out of every twenty-five Caucasian adults is a carrier of CF—that is, has a single copy of one of the CF gene mutations; two copies are required to develop the disease. One out of every three thousand live white infants will be diagnosed with CF. CF is a multisystem illness characterized in part by recurrent pulmonary infections, an inability to absorb dietary fat, and male infertility. Most children with cystic fibrosis will progress to respiratory failure, the average age of death being twenty-nine years. CF is principally diagnosed by a sweat test that examines the sodium and chloride in the sweat.[7]

BEGINNING THE STORY: MAKING THE DIAGNOSIS

A family may remember the day a child is diagnosed with CF as the day the dream of a healthy family evaporated. That day changes the entire family forever, since a positive diagnosis for the child means that both parents are carriers, other children in the family may also have CF, and all future children have a 25 percent chance of having CF and a 50 percent chance of being a carrier. So the diagnosis foretells not just the premature death of *this* child, but also the death of the dream of a certain kind of family, a threat to this and all ongoing generations.

When I was completing my training, the gene for cystic fibrosis had recently been discovered.[8] At that time we were taught to tell parents that life with cystic fibrosis would be radically transformed by gene therapy. We were taught to tell parents that their child's life would be a new story of technological rescue, and we were told to discard the old story of chronic illness and premature death. We were told to tell parents not to worry, since the cure was around the corner: CF would soon be conquered by progress.

Was this optimistic stance the best choice? In a principlist account of ethics, we might reason that the primary ethical duty of the physician in this instance is to act as an accurate conduit for knowledge so as to enhance the autonomy of the parents. The obligation to do no harm might lead physicians to temper their enthusiasm for still unknown therapies. Yet viewing the physician's ethical duty in these terms fails to address the temptation to paint a bright future and ignores the ways in which the situation plays into both the internal fantasies of the physician and the desperate fears of the parent. In this way, this view fails to account for the narrative structure of ethics.

A simple principlist approach would ignore the underlying narratives, fail to ask who else is in the room, fail to acknowledge the effect of the diagnosis on the past and future understanding of the family as a whole, and fail to see the sweat test result as something with far-reaching implications, something more than a straightforward test result. In contrast, a narrative approach prompts us to ask, "Who are the characters in this drama? Who is present but unseen?"[9] Ought the doctor to present himself as the rescuer, and if so, does his heroism constrain the family's response? What is the good parent supposed to do with this news—weep or sing praises to progress?

Narrative thinking allows physicians to perceive what is not stated, to put their work and words into the context of a family's life, and to live up to the moral duties enshrined in ethical principles with sensitivity and compassion. Unfortunately, the narrative of rescue is seductive. It not only permits the doctor to avoid being a harbinger of death but also allows the family to cement over the threat to its life story with a thick layer of hope. The consequences of such over-whelming hope can be brutal.

An eleven-year-old girl with CF had a sharp decline in her respiratory func-tion and over three months became increasingly debilitated and bed-bound. She was desperately weak and not responding to any of the usual therapies. Her death appeared imminent. Her parents had believed the rescue stories and had expected their child to live until the cure became available. Their fury at the physicians was expressed in shouting matches in front of the child, "You said she wouldn't die until she was thirty! What about the years of life you owe us? Do something!" The girl died after a hurried, painful, and self-consciously futile attempt to "work her up for a lung transplant" in the intensive care unit, gasping for air, blue in the face, because her parents believed the doctors' story that the cure was at hand. This message was first given when she was diagnosed as an infant, perhaps in an awk-ward attempt to keep tragedy at bay, or perhaps in a well-meaning attempt to sub-stitute hope for despair. But the process of creating narratives for others is messy: rather than portray a realistic and uncertain view of the trajectory of the child's life as time went on, we physicians had continued to collude with the parents in a story of heroic rescue by technology. We had not left room for other stories of the child's life, stories that could include uncertainty, or a sense of the preciousness of the present or the harm of unnecessary suffering. The family could see only one future: progress would rescue them. So tragedy caught them by surprise, and the story they now tell of their child's death is "we waited too long to get her on the transplant list."

How could things have gone better for this family and this child? We might have recognized that we, and the family, were believing too strongly in our mes-sages of progress. We might have recognized that the family had no story in reserve, no narrative other than what we had instilled in them, a constant and ever vigilant fight against disease. We might have recognized the hopeless outcome of such overweening faith in medicine. We might have recognized it, that is, had we not been adherents of the same faith.

From the point of view of a more traditional ethics, there is no error in this case, for the parents were the appropriate surrogate decision-makers, and they were making what they viewed as the appropriate decisions for their child. But from the narrative point of view, the death of this child was doubly tragic, for the physicians and the parents were caught up in a rescue fantasy that precluded preparation for the possibility of death, discounted the current suffering of the child in favor of an unrealistic future, and supplanted a child's story with a story about the failures of her parents and her doctors.

ENDING THE STORY: A MATTER OF CHOICE

Prior to the 1990s, the usual scenario of death from CF was progressive respira-tory failure, with death occurring on the hospital ward or at home.[10] Only very rarely were CF patients placed in the intensive care unit, as the use of a mechanical ventilator in a patient with CF was considered to be the paradigm case of prolonging death; no patient would want it and no compassionate doctor would offer it.[11] In short, the use of a ventilator for patients with CF was thought to be unethical because it was the perfect example of futile medical care.

The advent of lung transplantation in the early 1990s was a direct challenge to this noninterventionist consensus and had a profound effect on how all CF patients were to die. Patients on the transplant list began to be treated much more aggressively at the end of life than their similarly sick counterparts who had not opted for transplantation. Patients awaiting transplantation were placed on assisted ventilation by means of biphasic positive airway pressure, or "BiPAP," a newer method of positive pressure ventilation via a tightly fitting face or nose mask.[12]

The change in the consensus about aggressive care at the end of life affected even those patients who did not wish to be on the transplant list. Because doctors and patients were now more familiar with the methods of assisted ventilation and because their use in one type of CF patient now became acceptable, the use of BiPAP became a standard feature of the narrative of dying of CF.

A forty-one-year-old patient, a longtime survivor by CF standards, was having increasing difficulty breathing, and none of the usual treatments was giving him any sustained relief. He had long ago decided not to go on the transplant list and he was clear about not wanting to go to the ICU at the end of his life. His physician, familiar with the use of BiPAP for patients on the transplant list, offered him the choice of this new therapy.

The patient agreed to be placed on BiPAP when his breathing became labored and as the level of carbon dioxide in his blood rose higher and higher. Although his breathing improved on BiPAP, he was now dependent on the machine and deeply upset by this dependence. He had expected that his death would be gradual, with gradual onset of unconsciousness. This had been the norm for those patients dying before BiPAP was available. Instead, he could now survive, but only if he stayed tethered to the machine, and his death became, as he said, "up to him." He explained, "This machine has turned my death into a suicide. This has changed the story of my life." He must now choose to stay on the machine and live, or remove it and die.

How could we understand or respond to this man's anguish? What bothered him was having a choice, and yet it is exactly this presence of choice that is so valorized by the rescue narrative of the physicians—we heroes of high technology who saw the machine as having opened up a range of previously unavailable choices. The presence of choice is also a valued goal of much of traditional medical ethics. Yet for this patient, solace and meaning had been found in an inevitability, a *lack of choice* that formed the background of his character and his life. For him, knowing that he would die was not a source of suffering. He had framed himself as a survivor of CF and reveled in that success, even though he had been a heavy drinker and smoker. He had "beaten" CF (and medicine) at its own game by surviving longer than he "should have," and was now living to tell the tale.

But suddenly the tale had a different ending, an ending of enforced choice: live on the machine or die. No longer could he thumb his nose at the gods and dare them to kill him. Now he would have to *decide* to die. After several months on BiPAP, he was found dead at home by his visiting nurse, the machine disconnected but still at the bedside.

In one view of medical ethics, there was nothing wrong with this case: a competent patient was given a choice, and he made a decision. How could he, and how could we, have known the unintended consequence of his choice? Taking a narrative view helps us answer the question. We might have known if we had understood his life better, if we had been less seduced by our own need to rescue him and more attuned to a story whose expected ending had framed the plot of his life.

SOME CONCLUSIONS ON NARRATIVES IN PEDIATRIC PRACTICE

These cases demonstrate the often unseen influence of narratives in the care of seriously ill children. The pediatric narrative of rescue comes into conflict with other family-centered narratives and overwhelms other ways of making meaning out of life and death. The relentless pursuit of a cure by doctors and families is appropriate in many cases, but not in all. Sole reliance on the rescue narrative, by playing into the doctor's admittedly useful fantasy of heroism and by allowing a family to avoid grieving, leaves us with few resources when the rescue fails. Heroism ill-prepares us for the inevitable, and death can only be evidence of our failed heroics. Without a sensitivity to different narratives, we might see care at the end of life as a series of discrete puzzles, each of which is a choice and each of which has a solution. We would then miss the richly lived and human continuity of life and death. If we acknowledge the power of our own narrative of rescue, we will instead see how it can blind us to tragedy and deny patients and families comfort, hope, and meaning when a cure is not possible.

NOTES

1. I write from my experience as a subspecialty pediatrician in a large tertiary care referral center; the cases are real, although some of the identifying details have been changed to protect confidentiality. I will sometimes lapse here into a telling of the story that does not use the impersonal style of much of the writing in medical ethics but rather adopts a personal style that I hope will convey some of the sense of anguish and power of the cases.
2. I would call this the "simple efficiency benefit" of a narrative approach; seeing a patient history as a story being told just makes it easier and faster to get the entire history.
3. I leave open whether this translating is faithful or accurate. The point is that seeing the patient's report as a story rather than as answers to a predetermined set of questions leads to a more efficient transfer of information for the physician, and acts as an inter-

nal organizing template for further questions. The recognition that a patient history is a story is a (commonly unnoticed) epiphany in a medical student's transition from student to doctor.

4. It is not only physical characteristics that are expressed along generational lines in families: we may be warned not to turn out like Uncle Joe, living a life of regret, but instead to be like Great-Grandmother, who was always kind to the neighbors.

5. The quotation marks are intentional. Parents usually say, "The child will die after the ventilator is removed," whereas pediatricians and ethicists almost uniformly say, "The child will be allowed to die after the ventilator is removed." The different locutions are interesting, in that the "allowed to" implies that the pediatricians still reserve the power to save the child, whereas the parents see death as happening without the involvement of the doctors. In light of the great linguistic lengths that doctors will go to in order to point out that the disease is the cause of death, not the removal of the ventilator, the persistence of the "allowed to die" phrase is somewhat puzzling. It likely reflects the asymmetry between the wish to take credit for any rescue and the avoidance of any responsibility for death.

6. Remember that many of the members of the ethics committee work in a pediatric hospital setting and so share the common rescue narrative about their work. An essential part of any ethics consultation is therefore the voice and presence of others for whom the rescue narrative is not so strong: family members who have had children with serious illnesses and members of the community who can see outside the traditional boundaries of pediatric practice.

7. Because of the elevated salt in the sweat, infants and children with CF taste salty when kissed.

8. For more about the CF gene, see James Brody, "Discovery of the Cystic Fibrosis Gene: The Interface of Basic Science and Clinical Medicine," *American Journal of Respiratory and Cell Biology* 1 (1989): 347–48.

9. Some possibilities are the other living children, future children, grandparents who also were carriers, relatives who died unexplained childhood deaths that are now explained. These unseen but present ancestors are marvelously described (for a different illness) in Selma Fraiberg's chapter "The Ghosts in the Nursery," in *The Magic Years: Understanding and Handling the Problems of Early Childhood* (New York: Scribner and Sons, 1959).

10. For more on end-of-life care in CF, see Walter Robinson, "Palliative Care in Cystic Fibrosis," *Journal of Palliative Medicine* 3 (2000):187–92; and Walter Robinson, Sophia Ravilly, Charles Berde, and Mary Ellen Wohl, "End of Life Care in Cystic Fibrosis," *Pediatrics* 100 (1997): 205–9.

11. This consensus was not based on evidence; a single paper (Pamela Davis and Paul DiSant' Agnese, "Assisted Ventilation for Patients with Cystic Fibrosis," *Journal of the American Medical Association* 239 [1978]: 1851–54) examined the use of the ventilator in patients with CF and concluded that there were clearly some patients who could survive for more than a year following brief periods of mechanical ventilation. The story of how the ethical consensus not to use ventilators developed, even in the face of the increasing use of ventilators in other chronic illnesses like muscular dystrophy, is not simply a story of advancing technology.

12. BiPAP is euphemistically called "noninvasive" ventilation, only because it does not "invade" the windpipe with a tube. Yet for most patients BiPAP invades their lives, as

they are connected to a machine that prevents eating, drinking, speaking sentences, or leaving the bedside. One patient described BiPAP as "a mechanical squid sucking on my face" (Bob Flanagan, *The Pain Journal* [San Francisco: Smart Art Press, 2000], 127). Thus the narrative of ordinary life collides with the rescue narrative of medicine: BiPAP is noninvasive from the doctor's point of view also because it is "not half as bad" as what is ordinarily done to patients.

CHAPTER 11

BEYOND THE AUTHORITATIVE VOICE: CASTING A WIDE NET IN ETHICS CONSULTATION
SUSAN B. RUBIN

T his chapter outlines ways in which narrative methods can be useful in guiding the critical first step in ethics consultation—constructing the description of the case. Knowing what information to gather, how to gather it, and how to interpret it are all essential parts of the skill and art of ethics consultation. Narrative methods, with their attention to issues of narrative frame, voice, and interpretative skill, can help ensure that information is gathered and interpreted in an appropriate and competent fashion. Narrative methods can sharpen our attunement to issues of how the narratives of a case or ethical dilemma are constructed, whose voices are given authority, which plot lines are considered relevant, and which possible resolutions are given consideration. And finally, narrative methods can provide the necessary foundation for the normative work that follows.

As I reflect on how I structure ethics consultations, I am struck by the powerful contribution narrative methods have made, and by how incomplete or problematic my consultations would have been without the steady influence of a narrative approach.[1] I am cognizant too that, while I make active use of narrative methods, I do not rely on them exclusively, particularly when it comes to engaging ethics committees in the hard work of normative reflection once the stories and stakeholders are gathered together in one room. From this experience I have learned that while narrative methods have much to contribute at the descriptive level of ethics consultation, their application at the normative level may be more limited. In what follows I will trace the influence narrative methods have had on my approach to ethics consultation and describe both the use to which narrative methods can be put and the resistance there may be to employing them.

My practice is structured according to the belief that ethics consultation is performed best when it is nested in an ongoing moral community dedicated to creating and holding open the moral space necessary for genuine reflection and discourse.[2] Rather than delegating the task of ethics consultation to a single "expert" or to a small group of dedicated individuals,[3] I advocate the model of a full, diverse, and broadly constituted ethics committee collaborating with an ethicist to do case consultations[4] using a thorough intake process and a deliberate methodology for the case consultation meeting.[5] I serve on committees that have worked together over time to develop a sense of moral community in which diverse perspectives are expected, welcomed, and honored and in which there is, consequently, a safe environment for genuine moral discourse. These committees have learned to ask pointed questions that draw out the complexity of cases, to be attuned to the dynamics of a consult as it unfolds, and to speak the truth skillfully and honestly in the presence of all of the stakeholders, including the patient, family or close intimates, and members of the health care team.

When a request for ethics consultation is made, the ethics committee chairs or intake teams composed of ethics committee members conduct an intake to gather preliminary information about the case and to make an assessment about whether ethics consultation is appropriate, that is, whether there is a genuine ethical dilemma. It is at this first stage in the consultative process, the intake process, that narrative methods are first employed. Every effort is deliberately made to cast the widest possible net in gathering information and giving all those involved in the case an opportunity to share their perspective and participate in the description of the dilemma.

This means that while the individual who has requested the consultation may provide the first rendition of the case story—unavoidably framed according to how he or she sees the case and what he or she finds problematic or challenging—the process does not end there. As part of the intake process, information and input are also sought from the patient, if he or she is well enough, the patient's family or close intimates as appropriate, and members of the health care team from all shifts, such as physicians, consultants, nurses, nurse's aides, respiratory therapists, social workers, case managers, and chaplains. Stakeholders are invited to share their perspectives on the dilemma, to provide background information, to fill in gaps in the story, to make corrections, and, in essence, to act as active authors and editors of the evolving narrative.

Inevitably the intake process uncovers widely divergent, even contradictory, stories about the same case. The physician says the patient is unresponsive, while the night shift nurses describe tender conversations they have had with the patient about treatment preferences; the day shift says that the patient has no family, while the evening shift reports regular family visits; the intensivists tell us the family is in denial, while the family members talk of the deep and abiding faith that is guiding them; the nurses report that everyone is in agreement with the plan for extubation, while the respiratory therapists report significant reservations. The list goes on.

Though the impressions and perspectives we uncover in the intake process may appear to be in stark contradiction to each other, it is almost never because the involved individuals are deliberately attempting to mislead us. Rather, it is because each individual develops impressions based on the elements of the case with which they are familiar, and unavoidably there are parts of the story they simply do not know. In this way, each individual can claim to hold only a piece of the story. By casting a wide net in the intake process, a mechanism is created for first gathering and piecing together all of the potentially disparate stories and then identifying the points on which there seems to be agreement and disagreement. This allows cases to emerge in all of their complexity, rather than permitting them to be described and filtered through the single lens of the individual who has requested the consultation.

There are several essential assumptions built into the use of such an intake process. First is the recognition that there is no one single "real" story of any case but many ways of seeing and telling the story. Second is the acknowledgment that perceptions about whether there is even an ethical dilemma, what that dilemma is, what factors are relevant to understanding the dilemma, and what possible resolutions might be appropriate are all influenced by one's position in relation to the case. When it comes to describing an ethics case, there is no "view from nowhere."[6] Each perspective is situated and each is necessarily incomplete. Last is the understanding that, when we engage in ethics consultation, we are just as actively engaged in constructing narratives as we are in pondering their appropriate resolution. Our construction of the narratives should therefore be just as much the subject of critical scrutiny as our normative recommendations.

My experience of the way cases unfold in the consultation process leads me to strongly discourage the seemingly widespread practice of offering what have been called "curbside consultations." In a typical curbside consultation, the person seeking advice presents his or her account of a case, and the narrative effectively stops there, thereby privileging the chosen perspective and narrative of the person requesting advice. The obvious problem with curbside consultations from a narrative perspective is that they are inevitably based on an incomplete telling of the story of a case and invariably fail to consider the full range of moral perspectives at stake. Taking the time to really work through a case from the intake process through the full committee case consultation rather than falling prey to the temptation to rush to judgment helps ensure that the advice given in an ethics consultation is the product of a thorough, inclusive, and defensible process.

Rather than rendering an opinion on the spot, the task of those conducting the intake is simply to gather information and assess whether the referral is appropriate—in other words, if there is an ethical dilemma. Once the intake process is accomplished, a meeting of the ethics committee is convened to which the patient (if well enough), the patient's close family and friends, along with all of the physicians, nurses, and other staff involved in the case are invited and in which they are encouraged to actively participate.[7] At the ethics committee meeting, stakeholders have an opportunity to tell their story in their own voice and to hear firsthand and respond to the story as told from the perspectives of the other stakeholders. In a significant way, the ethics committee becomes the interpretive community that is actively involved in the task of reading, hearing, and responding to the array of stories as they unfold.

It is in the presence of these narratives that the normative dimensions emerge. And it is at this level, once all the stories are gathered together, heard, and interpreted, that narrative tools are insufficient. What is needed at this point is not simply a description of what is or might be the case, but a consideration of what

normatively ought to be the case. In fact, that is one of the most significant contributions ethics consultation can make: thoughtful reflection and conversation
about the "ought" questions and the range of possible responses, all against the
backdrop of value uncertainty or value disagreement. The face-to-face encounter
of stakeholders, each taking responsibility for telling his or her own story, having
the opportunity to listen to and respond to other versions of the same story, and
having the benefit of the ethics committee's input pushes the discussion to this
next level.

But it is not enough to create the scene and the opportunity. The ethics committee has a responsibility to ensure that during the meeting there is an opportunity to hear the various stories about the case, to reflect on the moral appeals at
stake, to consider possible options that could be recommended, and to hear each
committee member's considered opinion of what the right or good act is given
their knowledge of and reflection on what has been uncovered in the consultation
process. Structuring and facilitating the conversation at this point to ensure the
opportunity for this kind of discussion is essential and is ultimately what distinguishes an ethics case consultation from a casual albeit interesting exchange.

The goal is not necessarily to achieve consensus or to "fix" the problem but
rather to heighten awareness of the nature, source, and reason for the moral disagreements that gave rise to the conflict, to provide a safe forum for the full hearing of the arguments on all sides of the dilemma, and to offer a range of normative
perspectives on the dilemma. The ultimate "product" of ethics consultation
becomes the conversation and spoken reflection of the committee in light of the
stories the stakeholders have brought and the story that unfolds in their communication with each other and the committee. In carefully structuring the conversation, the committee can ensure that each of the stories is not only heard but
thoughtfully reflected upon.

It is the task of the ethics committee as both an interpretive and moral community to consider the range of possible endings to the narrative that could be
recommended in light of what they have heard about the particulars of the case.
Approaching consultations in this way makes it clear that all narratives at every
stage in their development are constructed, and that there is no "one true" authoritative story in any ethics case. Rather, the ethics committee's task is to weave
together a series of sometimes conflicting stories, to give the power of constructing the telling of each story to those whose story it most fundamentally is, and
together to consider the best way of moving forward. One of the outgrowths of
the narrative approach is that it entails the sharing of power: the power of telling the story, commenting on it, revising it, and concluding it. Closure comes out
of the collective hearing and telling and responding to one another.

Despite the value of structuring ethics consultations in this fashion—avoiding curbside consultations, using a clear intake process, casting a wide net to
gather all the relevant information, inviting all stakeholders to participate, involving the full committee in consultations, and using a structured case consultation

methodology—ethics committees sometimes resist approaching ethics consulta-tion in this fuller way.

For example, the desire to be perceived as a clinically useful and responsive service can tempt ethics committees to convene on demand without having done an adequate intake or without even assessing whether the consultation is appro-priate. This practice can exclude significant information and individuals, thereby preventing the committee from offering a meaningful consultation grounded in the actual facts of the case. In order to determine that a genuine ethical dilemma is present and if so to gauge its dimensions, the ethics committee needs to gather sufficient information, identify the relevant stakeholders, and include all stake-holders' perspectives in the discussion.

Even if ethics committees support using a comprehensive intake process, casting a wide net, and involving all of the stakeholders in the process, some have a practice of meeting in closed session first before inviting the patient or family into the room. Inexperienced committees may lack confidence in their ability to hear or respond to the story of a case in real time and in all its messiness. They may want to ask pointed questions outside of the family's presence. They may want to be forewarned of any hidden dynamics of a case in order to properly interpret information that may or may not be publicly stated during the consulta-tion. Or they may feel a need to establish a common lens through which the nar-rative will be interpreted.

Whatever the reason, having a pre-meeting in which the involved health care professionals are given the privilege of owning and telling the story of the case sets up an inevitably biased process in which the ethics committee's allegiance is sub-tly established at the outset. This practice sends the unfortunate message that the involved health care professionals and the committee are all in agreement and have the "real" story of the case. When the family or other stakeholders are then invited in, they are at a real narrative disadvantage.

Appealing to a narrative frame of reference can highlight these sorts of defi-ciencies in the process of case consultation and point the way toward effective remedies. An ethics committee that takes seriously the insights of a narrative approach will find fault with practices that give certain stakeholders but not oth-ers the power to be the authoritative storytellers. While narrative methods can make important and corrective contributions to the ethics consultation process, ensuring that all stakeholders are given an opportunity to share their perspective on equal footing, applying narrative insights is not always as straightforward as it may seem.

A recent case from a hospital in which I consult illustrates other kinds of resistance there might be to using such methods. In this case, the ethics committee received a request for consultation from a reproductive endocrinologist who had reservations about providing assisted reproduction to a sixty-year-old patient. In responding to the request, the committee was faced with several classic choices that go to the heart of the viability and desirability of using narrative method.

First, the ethics committee chair could have called the physician back and offered an opinion about the dilemma, as seems to be standard practice in a number of medical centers. Alternatively, the physician could have been invited to present the case to the committee, without notifying or inviting the other stakeholders, another common practice. Neither of these options was seriously entertained. But, there was still resistance to following the complete ethics consultation model I have outlined above.

Some members of the intake team wondered whether it might be more appropriate for the ethics committee to respond to the consultation request by simply convening a meeting in which the general question of postmenopausal pregnancy would be discussed, independent of this specific case. Certainly there would be no shortage of questions to discuss: Is there an unfettered right to reproductive freedom at any age? Do physicians ever have a duty to accede to their patient's wishes even if they have reservations? Is it discriminatory to question the propriety of a sixty-year-old woman parenting while we frequently celebrate the virility of older men who impregnate their considerably younger partners? Should there be age limits set for the use of assisted reproduction as a matter of policy?

Several arguments were presented in favor of having a "purely" theoretical discussion of the issues surrounding postmenopausal pregnancy instead of a specific discussion of this particular case in the presence of and with the participation of all of the stakeholders. The intake team did not want to unwittingly set up a dynamic in which the patient might be led to falsely believe that the committee was a tribunal in front of whom she was to plead her case. But there was a deeper reservation as well. Some members of the intake team feared that inviting the patient to the meeting might lead the committee to focus on the idiosyncratic features of her case that might or might not be relevant to the ethical analysis or, to put a finer point on it, that might lead the committee to treat her case differently or partially.

This reservation goes to the heart of the ambivalence practitioners may feel in incorporating narrative methods in ethics consultation. Narrative draws our attention to the particular, but is the particular relevant, and, further, is it fair to be swayed by the particular when engaged in an ethical analysis? In other words, does embracing a narrative approach inherently violate our time-honored commitments to fairness, justice, and impartiality?[8]

In response to these concerns, and drawing on a narrative approach, I argue that our attempts at abstraction are inevitably and unavoidably influenced by the typically unacknowledged lens through which we view any ethical dilemma. The virtue of deliberately using a narrative approach is that it forces us to expose our assumptions and biases, to confront them, and to bring competing allegiances into dialogue with one another. In so doing, it draws our attention to the morally relevant particulars of each case and our relation to them. Narrative methods contend that it does make a difference who the stakeholders are and how they see the dilemma, it does make a difference what their position is and their reasons are for taking that stance, and these particulars ought to make a difference in our analysis.

Interestingly, the American Society of Reproductive Medicine's position statement on oocyte donation in postmenopausal pregnancy similarly acknowledges the importance of attending to the particulars of each case and ultimately urges a case-by-case analysis rather than a categorical decision for or against postmenopausal assisted reproduction.[9] Once the intake process was invoked in this case, we had an opportunity to gather more information from not only the physician's but also the patient's perspective. We learned that this patient was significantly older than the age limit this physician had set as a matter of his office policies. We learned that the patient had recently entered into a second marriage with a man twenty-five years her junior, that she had three adult children, one of whom was only a few years younger than her new husband.

After gathering further information and concluding that there was a genuine ethical dilemma, the intake team called a full meeting of the ethics committee to which the patient and her husband and the relevant members of the health care team were invited. At the beginning of the meeting we explained, as we do in every case consultation, that we would first review the information that had been gathered on intake, invite the stakeholders to add any additional information or clarification, and give the committee an opportunity to ask questions. We would then move to a consideration of the moral appeals at stake in the case and an exploration of the possible options that could be pursued. And finally, we would ask the committee members to offer their recommendations with a specific emphasis on the factors that influenced them, their reasoning, and their justification for their recommendations.

During the case consultation meeting, as frequently happens, the case narrative unfolded in still further ways, revealing more about the intentions, motivations, and concerns of each of the stakeholders. We learned that the patient had considered the option of surrogacy but specifically wanted the experience of being pregnant and bearing a child with her new husband. We learned that there was nothing she would rather do in the second part of her life than start a second family. We learned that she came to this decision after praying about it and that she planned to have several more children. We learned more about the patient's husband and how important it was to him to father a child with his new wife. We learned that they had a strong support system and extended families who were enthusiastic about the prospects of the couple getting pregnant. We also learned that the patient's own father had had his last child at age sixty-five with a wife twenty-five years his junior.

We learned more about the physician's concerns at the meeting as well, particularly his concerns about the cost to the medical group if there were complications and his concerns about his reputation among his peers if he agreed to offer assisted reproduction to this patient. We learned that the high-risk perinatologist could find no medical reason to refuse this patient's request, explaining that she was not at a particularly high risk for complications, and that if they developed, any complications could likely be routinely handled. We learned that another woman had recently contacted the physician to request assistance with post-menopausal pregnancy.

The committee listened, raised questions, offered a range of perspectives, and in the end called on each committee member to argue for the recommendation he or she found most persuasive. Most committee members were struck by the fact that we were not hearing an argument on medical grounds against the use of assisted reproduction. If there was no compelling medical reason to deny treatment, the overwhelming sense was that it would be unreasonable to set limits based on our own potential discomfort with this woman's choice. At the same time, some committee members noted that the physician had a right to refuse to provide a service that he found ethically troubling. Still others stressed the obligation we had to consider the best interest of the potential child or children and not only the rights of the patient or the physician. In the end, in this case as in any other, the final decision about the next steps was left with the stakeholders, since the goal of ethics consultation is to give the stakeholders new ways of thinking and talking about the dilemma they are facing, not to supplant the decision-making process. We subsequently learned that the physician ultimately agreed to honor the patient's request, and though they initially had trouble finding an egg donor who would agree, they are now proceeding. In addition, the physician's network is developing a policy setting an age limit for assisted reproduction and has asked the physician to not offer this option again.

A central contribution of this and all case consultation meetings is the opportunity it creates for all participants to speak, to be heard, and to be responded to both by each other and by an actively engaged ethics committee. Creating a forum for this kind of exchange is one of the most important contributions an ethics committee can make. It is also at this juncture that ethics committees can falter if they do not know what to do with all of the information that is shared or if they are unskilled in moving from a descriptive to a normative discussion. For example, in this case some committee members questioned whether the particulars of this woman's life as presented ought to make a difference to the ethical analysis of the case and, if so, which particulars were relevant. Other committee members noted the power of our own biases and our own susceptibility to being swayed by factors that may or may not be relevant. One concern that was voiced, for example, was the degree to which we might have been swayed by the patient's powerful telling of her story, especially since she was someone with whom most members of the committee could easily relate. As a white, middle-class, articulate, poised professional woman, she may have succeeded in making a more favorable impression than someone who was unlike most members of the committee. This possibility left open the question of how her case might have been heard differently if she was, for example, a poor woman of color, or an angry, volatile person.

The committee's reservations in this case remind us that part of the normative work of ethics committees is to explicitly evaluate which if any of the particular facts of a case ought to make a difference from an ethical perspective. For example, was it relevant that the patient's own father had a child late in life with a younger partner? Or that the physician had real concerns about his professional reputation among his colleagues? In answering these questions, it is critical to note the tendencies we might have to credit or discredit particular narratives and plot lines when they are held in relation to each other and to be aware of our own relationships to the stories as they unfold. The reservations that emerged in this case also underscore the importance of having a diverse committee that represents a wide range of perspectives, is committed to giving everyone a voice, and takes seriously its collective responsibility to be a fair and thoughtful interpretive community. Finally, using a rigorous methodology to structure the conversation and insisting that committee members offer justifications for their recommendations rather than merely stating their opinions elevates ethics consultation beyond a mere emotive exchange about an interesting collection of stories.

While narrative methods cannot do the work of ethical analysis alone, they can make important contributions to the process and outcome of ethics consultation, reminding us that all case narratives and descriptions of ethical dilemmas are constructed, revealing that there is no one authoritative voice and no one "real" story to any ethics case, stressing the importance of giving each stakeholder the power to tell his or her own story, and emphasizing that our task is to uncover, hold in tension, interpret, and respond to the range of stories that surround every case. Using narrative methods competently takes practice and involves learning new and perhaps unfamiliar skills. And it can be challenging to respond to the resistance that may emerge to implementing core insights of a narrative approach. But in the end, I am convinced that the field of ethics has much to learn and the practice of ethics consultation stands to significantly benefit if narrative insights are systematically incorporated, taught, and used as a core and accepted methodology.

NOTES

1. A few words about my professional background will provide a context for the rest of my comments. After completing my doctoral education in philosophy and bioethics, I joined the Bioethics Consultation Group (BCG), an ethics consulting firm, as a staff ethicist. Working at BCG gave me an unusual breadth and depth of clinical ethics experience. Together my colleagues and I helped to develop ethics programs in hospitals and to set up, train, and support the ongoing work of ethics committees in a variety of health care settings, including the national Kaiser Permanente system. It was at BCG that I first worked with Dr. Laurie Zoloth, with whom I later cofounded The Ethics Practice, a firm devoted to providing ethics education, research, and clinical consultation. The way that I practice ethics consultation today is substantially shaped by the experiences Dr. Zoloth and I have had over the years and the opportunities we have had to try out different methods and approaches to consultation in a wide range of settings. Together we developed the unique approach to ethics consultation outlined in this chapter.

2. Margaret U. Walker, "Keeping Moral Space Open: New Images of Ethics Consulting," *Hastings Center Report* 23 (March–April 1993): 33–40.

3. For a discussion of different models of ethics consultation see Judith Wilson Ross, "Case Consultation: The Committee or the Clinical Consultant?" *HEC Forum* 2 (1990): 289–98; and Michael D. Swenson and Ronald B. Miller, "Ethics Case Review in Health Care Institutions: Committees, Consultants, or Teams," *Archives of Internal Medicine* 152 (1992): 694–97.

4. For a discussion of different conceptions of the ethicist's role see Laurie Zoloth-Dorfman and Susan B. Rubin, "Navigators and Captains: Expertise in Clinical Ethics Consultation," *Theoretical Medicine* 18 (1997): 421–32.

5. For a discussion of consultation methodologies see Albert R. Jonsen, Mark Siegler, and William J. Winslade, *Clinical Ethics* (New York: Macmillan, 1982); *Forming a Moral Community: A Resource for Healthcare Ethics Committees* (Berkeley: Bioethics Consultation Group, 1992); and Franklin G. Miller, John C. Fletcher, and Joseph J. Fins, "Clinical Pragmatism: A Case Method of Moral Problem Solving," in *Introduction to Clinical Ethics*, ed. John C. Fletcher et al., 2nd ed. (Hagerstown, MD: University Publishing Group, 1997).

6. Thomas Nagel, *The View from Nowhere* (New York: Oxford University Press, 1986).

7. For a discussion of the role of the family in ethics consultation, see Gregory L. Stidham, Kate T. Christensen, and Gerald F. Burke, "The Role of Patients/Family Members in the Hospital Ethics Committee's Review and Deliberation," *HEC Forum* 2 (1990): 3–17; Susan Wolf, "Ethics Committees and Due Process: Nesting Rights in a Community of Caring," *Maryland Law Review* 50 (1991): 798–858; George J. Agich and Stuart J. Youngner, "For Experts Only? Access to Hospital Ethics Committees," *Hastings Center Report* 21 (September–October 1991): 17–24; Susan Rubin and Laurie Zoloth Dorfman, "First-Person Plural: Community and Method in Ethics Consultation," *Journal of Clinical Ethics* 5 (Spring 1994): 49–54; and John C. Fletcher, "Ethics Consultants and Surrogates: Can We Do Better?" *Journal of Clinical Ethics* 8 (Spring 1997): 50–59.

8. My thanks go to Dr. Jeffrey Burack for raising this insightful and important point.

9. American Society for Reproductive Medicine's Ethics Committee Statement on Oocyte Donation to Postmenopausal Women, 1996.

CHAPTER 12

OF SYMBOLS AND SILENCE: USING NARRATIVE AND ITS INTERPRETATION TO FOSTER PHYSICIAN UNDERSTANDING
MARCIA DAY CHILDRESS

E thical ways of being and doctoring depend on knowledge of human particularity that the physician is always acquiring through attentive observation and reflection. Knowledge so gained—about the patient, to be sure, but also about the doctor—is just as crucial to the physician's clinical excellence as his or her fund of medical knowledge, and, together with this medical knowledge, it becomes the basis for the physician's understanding, for action, and for care.

The practice of ethics in the context of clinical medicine is fundamentally a matter of attention and interpretation. In a narrative model of medicine, the patient-physician relationship is cast as an ongoing, constructive conversation leading first and most immediately to diagnosis, prognosis, and treatment. The physician is the "critical reader," highly skilled both in eliciting and interpreting the patient's "story," which encompasses all that the patient says, how he or she says it, and the myriad nonverbal cues (including body language, significant omissions, and broad lacunae of silence) that accompany this telling. The physician's responsibility is to listen to the patient in a close, careful, and nuanced way in order to elucidate and then explain the patient's narrative, bring out and reflect its coherence and meaning, and finally translate what the patient has said and enacted into the formulaic tale—the case presentation—with which clinical medicine works.[1]

In a narrative model of medicine, the ongoing patient-physician relationship itself becomes a means of continuing the physician's education. In medical school, we frequently tell students that their patients are, and will be, their greatest teachers. While this seems a sage pronouncement, it is unclear whether faculty physicians really believe it and to what extent they practice it years after being wide-eyed students. What might they be learning, about themselves and about doctoring, from their patients? And how might such learning occur? While a busy practice allows little time for the physician's reflective analysis of interactions with every patient, there are certain patients who, for whatever reason, preoccupy the physician. In a narrative model of medicine, these patients, through their storied exchanges with the physician, may become to the doctor "teaching cases," opportunities for the physician to learn about himself or herself. David Morris suggests that, although neither American culture generally nor medicine specifically has focused on this phenomenon, we do regularly "think *with* stories."[2] Thus it is that certain stories in the doctor's experience can exert a moral call and have a thoroughly transformative power, even to the point of "'making you want to replace yourself.'"[3]

In medical education and training, even if a narrative model of medicine is invoked along with the data-driven biomedical model, seldom, if at all, are students and residents taught the sorts of interpretive precepts and skills of close reading that will help them to make the most of the narratives that they hear and, in turn, construct. And yet such practical strategies can make the difference between the physician treating the patient's story *as adjunct to* the presentation of physical signs and symptoms and understanding it *as* that presentation, the verbal equivalent of a complex state of being—illness—that includes, but is not limited to, physical manifestations of disease or dysfunction.

Medical faculty can teach students to become meticulously attentive to the narratives they hear, to learn as much as they can about what is being conveyed in and by a patient's story, and then to interpret their findings. A story from my own experience teaching first-year medical students illustrates how one might use narrative and interpretive strategies in the teaching of physicians, young and old. This "case" shows how attention to and interpretation of patients' narratives help doctors to know patients better, to recognize and respect those patients' values, and also to become more self-aware as physicians.

A course required of all first-year medical students, "The Doctor, the Patient, and the Illness" (DPI), addresses the patient's experience of illness, medical interviewing, and the fundamentals of the patient-physician relationship. Much of DPI focuses on the narratives of actual and standardized patients, elicited and collected by students very new to interacting professionally with ill persons. Groups of six students met weekly with two faculty mentors, one a physician and the other a nonphysician acquainted with the medical setting and knowledgeable about human behavior and communication. Within each DPI group, pairs of students were assigned "longitudinal patients," persons with chronic health problems who were selected from the physician-mentor's own panel of patients. The students made three home visits to these patients during the year, never in the company of their mentors. After every visit, students wrote brief narratives describing their interactions; students read their narratives aloud to their group and discussed their visits. In the rich conversation that accompanied students' presentations, faculty preceptors had ample opportunity to foster and test the students' "critical reading" skills, to help them attend not only to what the patients said (often in direct response to the students' unwitting cues) and how and when in the interview they said it, but also to what they did not say and to what the patients may have meant by their words or, even, by their silences.

The actual events comprising this case, which unfolded over three years, proved to be a fine learning experience for the students in the DPI group and for

Dr. B., the physician with whom I taught DPI. In addition, years after the original occurrence, this case has also become important to cite in discussions—with students, residents, and faculty—about why narrative competence is integral to the doctor's knowing both patient and self. In transforming this case into a vignette for teaching, I talked first with the patient's family (the patient is now deceased) and secured their permission; I also received permission from Dr. B. to publish a report of this case. I changed names and details to protect privacy and preserve confidentiality.

KNOWING THE OTHER: RECOGNIZING THE SYMBOLIC IN THE PATIENT'S STORY

Mr. Chambers, a fifty-eight-year-old divorced gentleman farmer, lived alone on two hundred acres of rolling land first owned by his grandfather. Like his grandfather and father before him, he maintained apple and peach orchards. Two first-year medical students, Rob and Craig, were assigned to visit Mr. Chambers at home three times during the year, to talk with him about the impact on his life of his chronic medical conditions: long-standing insulin-dependent diabetes and, more recently, deteriorating kidney function. Rob and Craig wrote brief narrative accounts after each visit with Mr. Chambers and shared these with the DPI group.

Writing about their initial visit, Rob and Craig characterized Mr. Chambers as a man of few words, with even fewer words to offer about his health. They spent most of the time outdoors with him and his little dog, while he walked them through the orchards and regaled them with tales of his younger, wilder days on the farm. Indoors, with the dog asleep on Rob's lap, they talked about Mr. Chambers's illness, how he had recently learned that, within a year, he would likely be on dialysis and perhaps also seeking a kidney transplant. They heard him talk too about the life implications of his illness: how his life expectancy was likely less than five years, how his health insurance was due to run out in the next year, and how he was considering marrying his girlfriend, who lived and worked in Baltimore, but didn't wish to be a burden, financially or otherwise, as his health declined and substantial medical expenses loomed.

Preparing to depart, the students stopped, at Mr. Chambers's invitation, at a fenced pasture that flanked Mr. Chambers's driveway, just downhill from the house. He whistled, and a horse came galloping toward them from the far side of the field. This horse, he claimed, could toss sticks and play "catch" with itself. Born on the farm and never saddle-broken, the horse lived alone in the pasture, self-sufficient and too wild to be caught. Whistling again, Mr. Chambers pitched a stick into the pasture; retrieving it, the horse tossed it aloft, then chased after it.

In oral presentations after this initial visit, both students voiced frustration with Mr. Chambers's reticence. They had found it nearly impossible to extract from him specifics about his medical condition and its effects on his daily life. They felt they had little to show (or write about) for their time with him.

Interestingly, though, their written narratives told quite another story. Both students' papers about this first visit were remarkable for lengthy discussion of their encounter with the horse in the pasture. While the students felt that they had filled their required two pages with extraneous information—a description of the farm and the tale of the horse—they had actually, unwittingly, captured the heart of Mr. Chambers's story: the farm and the horse were Mr. Chambers's roundabout ways of presenting what he valued most. *They were his story.* The horse, indeed, seemed a symbol or metaphor for Mr. Chambers himself.

Hearing their stories, and hearing also how difficult it was to talk directly with the patient about his problems, I asked the students to pay special attention in upcoming visits to what transpired with the horse. In telling our own stories, even the least sophisticated among us uses metaphors and speaks in symbolic terms. A person's chosen symbols are oblique means of self-disclosure, often revelatory to a depth unacknowledged and unintended by the speaker. As Joanne Trautmann Banks acknowledges, "human beings create symbols and are, in turn, transformed by them."[4] The students should see what they could learn of Mr. Chambers by talking with him about the horse.

Arriving for their second visit on a bitter winter afternoon, Rob and Craig found the pasture empty. They figured the horse was in a barn, sheltered from the cold. But Mr. Chambers quickly explained: the horse had been sold. Mr. Chambers seemed at once proud and regretful. Even as he crowed that it had taken nine men and two hours to load the recalcitrant horse into the new owner's trailer, he seemed sorry he'd made the sale. He had done so, though, in anticipation of spending more time with his girlfriend, who had offered to care for him through either dialysis or a transplant, in Baltimore. Indeed, Mr. Chambers allowed that, with these prospective changes in mind and with growing fears about his deteriorating health, he was considering selling the farm.

The students' presentations about their second visit were all about the horse's absence, reflecting Mr. Chambers's conversation with them, which was, they said, quite animated and detailed. They brought significant questions to class: What did the sale of the horse mean? How did this event connect with Mr. Chambers's failing health? By selling the horse and then witnessing its fight to stay at its birthplace, was Mr. Chambers testing possibilities for himself?

We all have ways of discerning meaning in our own life predicaments and deriving from our own life circumstances the means to arriving at crucial decisions. Such a process of seeking meaning, which may be "rehearsal" for major life choices, is not entirely rational or analytical, nor is it always enacted literally, on the surface of one's life, in the full light of one's own awareness. Rather, it may be undertaken and worked through on a subtle, symbolic level. Our small group discussed this process as it seemed to be unfolding for Mr. Chambers. Understanding that he had earlier established significant parallels between himself and the horse, the students were inclined to see his sale of the horse, and his sadness in its wake, in this light.

The students' last visit, in the bloom of spring, brought news that Mr. Chambers had been quite ill, had begun dialysis, and was now listed for a kidney transplant. While still considering the sale of his property and the move to Baltimore, he had taken no definitive steps in this direction. The students' visit was pleasant but short and low-key. In their write-ups, Rob and Craig remarked on the empty pasture but noted that Mr. Chambers, preoccupied with how he was feeling, spoke of neither horse nor farm.

At year's end, reporting on their last visit, the students seemed disappointed; without the horse as reference point, conversation had flagged. The patient was once again fairly tight-lipped and, his health having slipped markedly, he seemed resigned and in something of a holding pattern about life decisions.

One early summer day two full years after Rob and Craig had made their visits, a small notice appeared in the local newspaper: "Man Drowns in Pond." Naming no names, the news brief identified a farm east of town where a sixty-year-old man had been reported missing from his bedroom in the early hours of the morning by his son and daughter-in-law; the next afternoon, his body was recovered from the pond in the pasture below the house.

An obituary for Mr. Chambers appeared in the paper later that week.

When Mr. Chambers died, our six DPI students were in their third year, scattered among clinical clerkships. Dr. B. and I sent them the news article and the obituary together with a note reminding them of how they had learned, through the saga of the proud, feisty horse, what mattered most to this gentleman: his bond with the land and his independent life there, even in defiance of illness that threatened to control his life. In the end, he had rejected the course he had rehearsed with the sale of the horse, choosing instead to remain on the farm, refuse remarriage, and take his own life before disease ravaged it further, "claiming," Dr. B. said, "his beloved land with his body."

KNOWING ONESELF: INQUIRING AFTER OUR OWN SILENCES

Dr. B., the physician-mentor with whom I taught DPI, was a senior professor of medicine with a sharp mind, agile wit, and gracious manner. He was well known in the medical school as a champion of his patients—he had legions of grateful patients—and also as something of a master storyteller. Educated and trained in the 1940s and 1950s, he was much more comfortable with a strictly biomedical and rather paternalistic model of medicine than with a broader, more egalitarian biopsychosocial model. A narrative model of medicine he never quite understood. Course guidelines to the contrary, with our students he equated the patient's story with the history of the present illness and the process of eliciting the story with that of taking the history. Whenever these differences became problematic in class, Dr. B. and I would discuss with our students generational disparities in ways of understanding and practicing medicine.

Just three months before we began teaching together, Dr. B. had closed a long, successful practice as an endocrinologist specializing in diabetes. He had been for many years Mr. Chambers's primary physician. Briefing the class, Dr. B. had reviewed Mr. Chambers's diabetes-associated problems, then mentioned that, on closing his practice, he had referred Mr. Chambers to a nephrologist rather than to another endocrinologist, because Mr. Chambers was already experiencing renal failure and would doubtless need either dialysis or a transplant within a few years. Rather sheepishly, he confessed that the timing of his retirement enabled him to deliver Mr. Chambers into the care of the appropriate subspecialist without *his* ever having to give Mr. Chambers the devastating news about his deteriorating condition.

As Rob and Craig's story of Mr. Chambers unfolded through the year, it had a profound effect on Dr. B. The patient he had known for years was revealed to him in new and poignant ways. Granted, he had always seen Mr. Chambers in the office, never on the farm; had seen him chiefly to monitor his diabetes and manage its complications; had seen him as a repository of clinical information and as the immediate object of his own medical ministrations. That is, he had seen Mr. Chambers within the constraints of the biomedical model, which revels in the patient's data but admits neither the patient's voice nor story, and which bids doctor and patient be silent about whatever lies beyond biomedicine's narrow ken. For Dr. B., Mr. Chambers in all his human complexity and proud symbolic identifications remained unknown, because not inquired after, until Rob and Craig, in their medically naïve narratives, discovered and introduced him.

The biomedical approach practiced for years by Dr. B. had structured his interactions with Mr. Chambers so that, underlying their factual exchanges and genteel banter, there prevailed between the two of them potentially problematic gaps or silences consisting of generous clinical distance and, at the last, on Dr. B.'s part, gentle deception. What Dr. B. discovered in the narrative approach practiced by our students was a way to know Mr. Chambers as a *subject*, to learn particulars of his life, to grasp his values, to gain insight into his choices. This narrative way of knowing so significantly augmented what he had known through the biomedical model that the seasoned clinician seemed stunned by the *proximity* and *nobility* of Mr. Chambers as presented by Rob and Craig. Dr. B. also seemed stunned by his own fondness for the man.

By the end of our DPI course, Dr. B. had come to understand and to speak of Mr. Chambers very differently than he had before. Significantly, two years later, when we together notified our students of the patient's passing, it was Dr. B. who chose the words—he "claim[ed] his beloved land with his body"—that explicitly recalled our narrative knowledge of Mr. Chambers and that voiced profound respect and love for this patient.

This story of Rob and Craig with Mr. Chambers (and Dr. B.'s story within the story) counsels physicians to listen for and attend to the metaphors and symbolic content in patients' narratives. It also encourages physicians, even experienced clinicians like Dr. B., to attend to what others' narratives may show them about patients whom they believe they know well. The story further urges physicians to inquire into their own significant silences in conversation with their patients for what they may learn about their own and medicine's resistances, fears, vulnerabilities, and defenses. By using narrative as a means of exploring areas formerly off-limits, they may also learn to cultivate a vocabulary within their medical lexicon for self-examination and self-reflection. What this approach accomplishes is nothing less than a radical revision in the doctor's way of being a physician.

But a caution: if thinking *with* stories is to contribute substantively to ethical ways of doctoring, physicians need considerable self-awareness as tellers and hearers of stories. They also need good interpretive skills with which to understand the myriad stories that fill their practice life. Typically, and certainly until recent years, medical schools have neither emphasized nor explicitly taught such skills. Enter humanities and, especially, literature scholars as medical educators. Such scholars, "who view the world through, and as, narrative," understand narrative ways of knowing self and other and, once acclimated to and conversant with the medical environment, can teach narrative interpretation and self-reflection as critical clinical skills.[5] As teachers in medicine, literature scholars can "read" clinical scenarios and the narrative characterizations of those scenarios; they then can challenge medical students and even faculty physicians to parse their clinical encounters, become attuned to their patients' voices, read critically the words and ways of their patients and themselves, excavate layers of meaning in the stories they hear and tell, and inquire after and interpret symbols and silences—in short, to practice medicine with narrative competence.

NOTES

1. Rita Charon, "Doctor-Patient/Reader-Writer: Learning to Find the Text," *Soundings* 72 (1989): 137–52; Kathryn Montgomery (Hunter), *Doctors' Stories: The Narrative Structure of Medical Knowledge* (Princeton: Princeton University Press, 1991); Howard Brody, "'My Story Is Broken; Can You Help Me Fix It?' Medical Ethics and the Joint Construction of Narrative," *Literature and Medicine* 13 (1994): 79–92.
2. David B. Morris, chapter 20 in this volume, 196.
3. Ibid., 197.
4. Joanne Trautmann Banks, chapter 21 in this volume, 221.
5. Ibid., 225.

CHAPTER 13

NARRATIVE UNDERSTANDING AND METHODS IN PSYCHIATRY AND BEHAVIORAL HEALTH
RICHARD MARTINEZ

INTRODUCTION

I n recent years, narrative approaches in clinical and ethical decision-making in psychiatry, psychotherapy, and behavioral health have increased in importance. While the waning of psychoanalytic and psychodynamic teaching in residency programs and the increased effectiveness of psychopharmacologic interventions in clinical practice have decreased the profession's reliance on interpretive or "talking" psychotherapy, the influence of the medical humanities has increased interest and curiosity about narrative theory and application in the behavioral health fields. Managed care has had a negative impact on health care education and health care practice, and yet it has had a positive impact by fueling new discussion and reflection upon the fundamental ethical aspects that define the patient-professional relationship in health care.

In this chapter, I present the case of J.S., a former patient who was in treatment with me for more than ten years and helped me to explore ways in which narrative can improve clinical and ethical decision-making in psychiatry and psychotherapy.[1] A narrative therapeutic approach evolved in our work together over the last ten years. J.S. has reviewed this manuscript and has given permission for its publication. I have changed several elements to protect her privacy.

THE CASE OF J.S.

J.S. is a forty-five-year-old divorced woman. Her first appointment with me was ten years ago. In those first sessions, she told me that she had seen another psychiatrist, Dr. A., who had diagnosed her with major depression, anxiety disorder, post-traumatic stress disorder, and a mild borderline personality disorder. She was treated with several medications, including an antidepressant, an antianxiety medication, and a medication for occasional sleep disturbance. Over the years, she had tried numerous antidepressants, antianxiety agents, and mood-stabilizing medications. At the time of her first visit with me, she believed that she was on an optimal combination of medications.

She had been in treatment with Dr. A. for about twelve years. She first came under his care when she had made an attempt on her life—she was twenty-three years old at the time—and was hospitalized for the first and only time in her life. Dr. A.'s retirement prompted J.S. to seek a new psychiatrist. During her initial visits with me, she was cautious, somewhat sad, and somewhat angry that she was being "forced" to seek another psychiatrist for treatment and the "management" of her medications. In the first two sessions, she told of her background and childhood, of her work and family situation, and of her past psychiatric treatment, including the hospitalization. Although the medications had brought some improvement in symptoms of depression and anxiety, she continued to suffer with occasional nightmares, complete sexual displeasure during her previous marriage and during all her past relationships with men, intermittent suicidal thoughts, and fear of further intimate involvement with men. Although feeling terribly lonely and estranged from members of her family, including her mother, she reported that her three children—ages seven, ten, and twelve when she first came to see me—were her main reason for not ending her life.

In our initial interview, she reported incoherent memories suggesting sexual abuse by her father. She believed that these memories suggested that some inappropriate sexual activity occurred with her father when she was between eight and eleven years old. Her father committed suicide when the patient was sixteen. J.S. believed that her father suffered with depression and, occasionally, psychosis. She worked as a social worker in a residential setting for teenagers with behavioral problems. She denied symptoms of mania or hypomania, denied psychotic symptoms although she reported some tendency to startle easily, and denied problems with drugs or alcohol. She had no guns or weapons in her home. At the time of her first meetings with me, she was sharing custody of her three children with her former husband, who had remarried. J.S. was the children's primary caretaker during the school year.

THE BIOPSYCHOSOCIAL PERSPECTIVE

The fields of psychiatry and psychotherapy are closely tied to the clinical and ethical traditions of medicine and the claims of medicine to care for the "whole patient." Many of the ethical issues relevant to general medicine are also important to the practice of psychiatry and psychotherapy.[2] Like medicine, psychiatry and related behavioral health fields are dominated by the biomedical model. The person seeking help is conceptualized as a "patient" inflicted with "disease" and deficient through "psychopathology." The patient presents the health care professional with a challenging riddle to be explored, described, and solved. Symptoms are data that support diagnoses. These symptoms are "targeted" by a "new generation" of psychopharmacological agents that calms these symptoms and treats the disease.

In 1977, psychiatrist George Engel proposed the biopsychosocial perspective as a theory to counter the emerging dominance of the biomedical model of theory and practice in health care.[3] Engel reminded medicine of its obligations to the whole patient, and he endorsed professional attention to emotional, social, and community dimensions of illness. Unfortunately, Engel's model has never had the influence in health care that many had hoped.

Although Engel's pioneering work warned of the dangers of reductionism in medicine and conceptualized a wide and integrated set of domains in which to consider a patient's illness, his framework was not designed to help clinicians understand the ethical or existential dimensions of patient assessment and treatment. An improvement over the preceding models for medicine, Engel's model stopped short of conceptualizing patients—and doctors—as singular individuals facing illness joined in intersubjective relationships. This help has come, since the mid-1980s, from the medical humanities, end-of-life care, and professional and medical ethics. A consensus is emerging that focuses medicine and its related fields on foundational professional obligations and responsibilities. These obligations and responsibilities include prevention of illness and injury and the promotion of health, understanding and alleviating suffering, providing comfort care to—and refusing to abandon—patients who cannot be rescued completely from the ravages of suffering and pain, and professional obligations to assist some patients who strive to make meaning of their illness experience.[4] As these new considerations eclipse some of the more traditional and mechanistic goals of medicine and psychiatry, the health professions are seeking frameworks more inclusive and robust even than Engel's with which to conceptualize their goals and try to reach them.

PSYCHIATRY AND MODERNISM

In the early 1980s, I was trained to believe that mental diseases, disorders, and conditions not only exist but are detectable, can be identified, and can be classified; when the proper targeted therapeutic interventions—psychopharmacologic, psychotherapeutic, or social—are administered, patients get better. Those patients who did not get better or did not get much better were thought to have either chronic mental disorders, such as schizophrenia or mood disorders, and/or personality disorders.

During this period, the developing biological view of the etiology and treatment of the mental disorders challenged the dominant psychoanalytic model, in spite of psychoanalysis's epistemological claim of legitimacy as a science.[5] Psychiatry and psychiatric nomenclature, including psychoanalysis, were joined to a medical model of knowledge, theory, and practice that continues to dominate the profession today. Beginning in 1989, anthropologist T. M. Luhrmann spent four years observing and interviewing psychiatric residents and other health professionals in various institutional settings across the country. She writes about the philosophic basis of today's psychiatry:

Psychiatrists have inherited the Cartesian dualism that is so marked a feature of our spiritual and moral landscape. Sometimes they talk about mental anguish as if it were cardiac disease: you treat it with medication, rest, and advice about the right way to eat and live.... When psychiatrists talk in this manner, psychosis and depression become likewise written on the body. This style of speaking has gained preeminence in the last two decades. It is usually called "biomedical" psychiatry, an approach to mental illness that treats it as an illness of the body that is more or less comparable to the other physical illnesses. Sometimes, though, psychiatrists talk about distress as something much more complicated, something that involves the kind of person you are: your intentions, your loves and hates, your messy, complicated past. This style is associated with psychoanalysis and psychoanalytic psychotherapy, usually called "psychodynamic.". . . From this vantage point, mental illness is in your mind and in your emotional reactions to other people. It is your "you."[6]

Like general medicine, psychiatry and related behavioral health fields are firmly established in a modernist scientific tradition, the culmination of the scientific method that arose from the Enlightenment view of knowledge and language. The positivist and analytic scientific method establishes the "truth" by reducing the objective and knowable world to its building blocks. Language is a nonambiguous, nonallusive, value-neutral description of this objective world. With the introduction of so-called designer psychiatric medications that supply or inhibit specific chemical neurotransmitters to the brain, biological interventions in mental disorders have become more predictably effective, at least for the short run. And with the increased efficacy of psychopharmacology, modernist beliefs and perspectives congruent with their use become all the more influential in psychiatric and behavioral health practices.

However, the modernist apparatus is insufficient to support the diagnosis and treatment of patients with mental disorders, because the solutions available through reductionist approaches, however effective they may seem at the time, do not alleviate the actual suffering witnessed in the sick. Proper identification, selection, and recommendation of optimal beneficial treatments for psychiatric disorders are necessary in order to deliver effective care. The central ethical dilemma facing the practice of psychiatry today—as well as the central professional and personal dilemma facing many practicing behavioral health professionals—is precisely to identify, select, and recommend the most beneficial mental health treatment for individual patients. If alleviating suffering, caring as well as curing, and not abandoning patients are central obligations and responsibilities, how can psychiatrists and other behavioral health professionals have confidence that they are fulfilling their ethical obligations to deliver optimal beneficial care, especially in the current financial and cultural environment, with only the instrumental methods of conventional treatment at their disposal? Although the biopsychosocial approach can increase that confidence, I believe it must be fortified by narrative knowledge and methods in order for today's psychiatry and other behavioral health practices to meet intellectual, professional, ethical, and existential duties toward the sick.

THE CASE OF J.S. REVISITED

The summary of J.S.'s condition and history reported above is similar to a case presentation that might be exchanged between two behavioral health professionals or between a supervisor and trainee. The language of this presentation is constructed in a way that highlights the pertinent biological and psychodynamic information necessary in order to determine justifiable interventions. Current and past medication interventions and the effectiveness of those medications along with a family history of potentially genetically linked mental conditions address biological causation and influences. Information about the patient's family; her past history, including pertinent childhood experiences; and her current subjective reports of how she is feeling and thinking provide a view of her psychological realm. Discussion of current symptoms and pertinent past psychiatric symptoms and treatment inform both the biological and psychological understanding of J.S. Lastly, information about her family life, work situation, and general information about relationships with others tell us about her social sphere. In the summary's brief and concise form as well as in its content, the biopsychosocial model is apparent.

Unfortunately, this biopsychosocial encapsulation of J.S. does not serve her fully. David Morris summarizes the deficiencies of the biopsychosocial approach. In *Illness and Culture in the Postmodern Age*, he offers three reasons to move beyond the biopsychosocial approach:

> First, its influence today is indirect at best, marginal at worst. Although a few medical schools make a biopsychosocial approach central to their teaching, elsewhere it is not so much opposed as treated with indifference or institutional cynicism. . . . Second, business as usual in crowded hospitals and clinics usually means drugs and surgery. There is little time for extensive psychosocial therapies, and the financial disincentives are strong. "Capitation fees". . . actively discourage focus on complex, nonbiological dimensions of illness. Third, and most important, the 1977 model that Engel called biopsychosocial needs significant revision in order to extend and enrich its understanding of cultural processes with the benefits of two decades of postmodern thinking.[7]

If psychiatry is committed to understanding and addressing the mental suffering of patients and to striving for optimal beneficial interventions, the biopsychosocial approach is inadequate. Morris's "biocultural" approach is an alternative. In this approach, narrative conceptual frameworks and methods are used to help psychiatrists and other behavioral health professionals tend to the patient's illness experience. A heightened reliance on narrative methods frees the clinician from the exclusive focus on the modernist preoccupation with disease.

In psychiatry, as in other medical specialties, ethical dilemmas arise out of the particulars of human drama. Narrative approaches allow attention to those detailed elements of language and storytelling that often are neglected in many psychiatric encounters. A narrative approach becomes a method for listening to and recognizing the moral dramas embedded in the clinical story. How can health care professionals provide guidance for ethical dilemmas if they do not have confidence in their perceptions and interpretations of their patients' problems and stories? Narrative becomes a tool that allows for penetration deep into the human moral drama that is involved in illness. Narrative methods help us to listen and see with intensified accuracy and reach—a hermeneutic stethoscope of a sort. Narrative improves our perception of the moral dilemmas and their complexity contained within all clinical encounters and can help us to focus on the ethical and existential elements involved in the care of those with mental suffering.

Empathy and compassion are given new life in the patient-professional relationship through narrative methods. Nontechnical language, close and attentive listening, and the professional's willingness to support the voice of the patient while resisting the psychiatric colonization of the patient's experience help to create this sphere of compassion and empathy. In his book *The Illness Narratives*, Arthur Kleinman offers a view of illness and suffering through the narrative lens. According to Kleinman, narrative brings order and cohesion to suffering. The health care professional helps the patient or family interpret suffering in the direction of meaning. The caregiver has the important task "to witness a life story, to validate its interpretation, and to affirm its value."[8] The narrative perspective allows for contextual understanding and illumination of the spiritual, existential, and cultural implications at work in the experience of illness.

THE CASE OF J.S. AND NARRATIVE

A biopsychosocial perspective encourages psychiatrists and other behavioral health professionals to think about and perceive patients and relationships with patients in a certain way. A narrative perspective encourages a different kind of clinical understanding of patients and of therapeutic relationships. With narrative, information about the biological and psychodynamic elements of a patient's story is only a component of the goals and purposes of the relationship. Certainly, psychiatrists and other behavioral health specialists need to know all of the information revealed through the biopsychosocial model. However, in addition to completing the checklist of information that supports biomedical and psychodynamic understanding, the psychiatrist or psychotherapist allows additional elements to emerge when he or she encourages the patient to tell her complete story. By hearing and acknowledging the patient's complete story, the behavioral health specialist accepts the obligations and responsibilities incurred by witnessing suffering. Caring and developing meaning-making relationships become therapeutic priorities. The patient-professional relationship is transformed both clinically and morally when the psychiatrist or psychotherapist begins to think, feel, and act through a narrative perspective. In the description below, I will try to answer several questions: How did a narrative approach change my work with J.S.? How did my perceptions, my listening, and my questions change as I worked in this narrative mode? How did narrative change my understanding and knowledge of J.S., and, thus, change my decisions and actions?

In the first sessions, I noted that J.S.—with twelve years of previous psychiatric treatment—was unusually adept at telling her story in a concise, summary form. I believed that this reflected J.S.'s many years of psychiatric treatment and familiarity with the dominant language and models of understanding in the behavioral health fields. She had learned to construct her story in the biopsychosocial format. In her first session, she provided a summary of her condition that could serve as a model for any behavioral health professional who wishes to perfect the biopsychosocial construction.

A narrative perspective in the early stages of assessment encouraged me to ask J.S. if she was satisfied with her summary and if there was more to her story. I reflected to J.S. that she was quite good at providing a concise summary and that she was familiar with the behavioral health field, but that she might have more to share or discuss. I pointed out that it seemed that it was important for her to begin her new relationship in a cooperative and joining spirit. I asked, "Why is it important for things to go well in the first interview?" J.S. spoke of some annoyance at changing psychiatrists. She was concerned that after twelve years with her previous psychiatrist, this change might not work. She was concerned that she might disappoint me. "Do you wish for our work together to be similar to or different from your work with Dr. A.?" I proceeded. "Were you afraid that I might change or not change your medications? What were your concerns about starting this new relationship? What were your fears and worries?"

In narrative, the psychiatrist provides a series of questions and listens carefully to responses as he or she undermines the usual expectation and dominance of the biological and psychodynamic conversation. The narrative method signals to the patient the important ethical value that the psychiatrist is interested in J.S. *as person* and is open to discuss and visit complex and diverse aspects of J.S. *as person* at the start of this new relationship. Immediately, I expressed my concern about her recent loss of her previous psychiatrist and demonstrated that I cared about her potential discomfort with a new psychiatrist, a total stranger. Through narrative methods, I quickly communicated that I wished to understand J.S. as a person who is suffering, a person who has had experiences in her life in which trust and respect have been compromised. After several years of therapy, J.S. told me that this approach in the early period of our relationship was extremely comforting during a time of great anxiety due to the change in psychiatrists. She was pleased to find a psychiatrist who was genuinely interested in her understanding of and experience with her difficulties and who respected her own interpretation of what she needed from a new psychiatrist.

The goals of the usual psychiatric or psychotherapeutic intake session—where questions are designed that help the behavioral health professional reach a diagnosis and recommend treatment—are made secondary in this approach. By acknowledging J.S. as a person who might subordinate her true voice in order to please and accommodate me, I encouraged J.S. to discover and exercise her own voice. Through narrative knowledge and practice, the psychiatrist encourages the patient to express her story and to reveal her important concerns and worries rather than to collude with the implicit power dynamics that are present in all first encounters between health care professionals and patients.

When J.S. talked of her medications and symptoms, she cooperated with the standard practice of privileging this information. A narrative method allows the psychiatrist to ask the patient not only about her own sense of the benefit of these medications, but to pose additional questions, questions that allow uncertainty and ambiguity to have legitimate value in the decisions regarding these interventions. Such a line of inquiry is intended to undermine the dominance of the biomedical model and to support the patient in a fuller experience of self-determination and decision-making authority. I asked J.S., "What do you think about taking medication? Do you feel this intervention is necessary or central to your wellbeing? How does it influence your sense of yourself as a person, as a mother? Do you have faith in the biological explanations of your conditions? What are your questions and doubts about medication? What are your frustrations with or confidence in this treatment approach?"

The narrative perspective supports the psychiatrist in disclosing his own thoughts and feelings about medication and its usefulness. I revealed to J.S. my own uncertainty and skepticism about the usefulness of medications for certain problems, while I reviewed what I knew to be the supporting literature about medication and its usefulness in situations similar to hers. A narrative approach supported this self-disclosure. The positivist biomedical model encourages health care professionals to limit expression about the inevitable uncertainties and ambiguities that are contained in all therapeutic interventions. In my early relationship with J.S., I approached interventions less authoritatively than I would have without the narrative perspective, and I supported the relationship as an enterprise in which mutuality and fairness are shared values. This is not "expert" speaking to "patient," but two persons struggling with complex problems and the difficult project of deciding and doing what will be useful and most beneficial for the patient.

Over the many years of our relationship, J.S. tried several medications that had not been available during her previous treatment. On two occasions, we agreed to ask for consultation from another psychiatrist who had greater expertise and experience in the use of psychotropic medication. J.S. found my willingness to use a consultant helpful. While her experience helped her to recognize the limits of medication, it was important to her that we not overlook possible benefits from new medications and new perspectives. Initially, she was concerned that I would abandon her if she sought the advice of consultants, that I might have seen this as a betrayal. After discussing this concern in numerous sessions and obtaining my support for the introduction of other perspectives in the management of her medication, J.S. expressed gratitude for my commitment to her, a commitment that encouraged other professional perspectives in the biological treatment of her depression and anxiety.

Suicidal thoughts and feelings are some of the most difficult considerations for many health care professionals. While it is clear that health care professionals cannot predict violence and suicide, most psychiatrists and other behavioral health professionals are trained to assess risks, and they have legal and ethical responsibilities to do so. While the discussion of "rational suicide" is common in the end-of-life care literature, there is little written on the subject of "rational suicide" and the psychiatric patient or client. Most behavioral health care professionals believe that their duty to assess risks and provide safety for their patients is more important than their duty to explore the deep moral and existential implications of suicide and suicidal thoughts.

In the case of J.S., suicidal thoughts—including at least one attempt on her life—were an important part of her story in the first session with me. Most of the information she provided helped me in the risk-assessment aspect of the early interviews. J.S. had made one suicide attempt in her twenties, currently suffered with chronic and recurrent suicidal thoughts, had no weapons immediately available to her, and reported that her children are a main reason for not acting on these feelings. In addition, J.S. told of her father's suicide, of her own current struggle with depression, and expressed the thought that suicide would be one remedy to her suffering. Biological and psychological aspects of the risk assessment are covered in this information.

How did the conversation about suicide with J.S. change when guided by the narrative approach? How did the conversation about "incoherent memories" of sexual abuse shift as I listened and understood, allowing the narrative paradigm to guide me? Respect for J.S. as a person assumed center stage. My duty to provide beneficial interventions, in part determined by the goals of medicine already discussed, guided my approach. J.S. was relieved to learn that I was interested in helping her understand her suicidal preoccupations while taking my responsibility for her safety seriously. At first, she was reluctant to probe the depth and quality of these feelings and thoughts. She explained to me the fear that if she "fully opened up about this," I would "put her in a hospital" and "take her children away." With my help, she was able to make some distinction between "thinking about suicide" and feeling frightened that she might "act on her fantasies." Over the years, as periods of despair became more manageable and better understood, her suicidal preoccupations waned. In recent years, she has expressed a "love" for living, a devotion to herself and her significant relationships, and a great sense of satisfaction that she was able to avoid her father's fate.

The principles of beneficence and respect for J.S.'s decisions could not have been realized without the process and quality of relationship supported through the narrative perspective. While certain goals of the biopsychosocial model were not abandoned, my narrative orientation supported specific values and approaches in the relationship with J.S. She was not only a person to be respected, but a person capable of and entitled to thoughts, feelings, and decisions that can be infinitely complex. At times, such thoughts, feelings, and decisions are beyond understanding. For example, J.S. was never able to "retrieve" specific memories of sexual abuse. While she gained confidence in the idea that "something inappropriate" occurred with her father, she learned to live with the uncertainty and incoherence of her memories. After many years of struggling to remember specific events or situations, she focused her efforts on the present. In a new and committed relationship that began several years ago, she has worked at transforming herself from an injured victim of her father's madness to a person building trust, allowing for the experience of love and a more satisfactory sexual relationship. At the time of this writing, J.S. continues to transform her father's legacy. I trusted J.S. to be the narrator of her own story. I agreed to join her in her story, to alter her story through my participation, but humbly to act in the recognition that I could never diminish J.S. in her own narrative experience and "storying" of her life.

POSTMODERN PSYCHIATRY

Unlike the biologic or psychodynamic perspectives embedded in the biopsychosocial approach, narrative transforms the process between patient and professional. Patients seek new meaning and understanding in their lives and relationships by "storying" their lives. As Michael White states in *Narrative Means to Therapeutic Ends*, "[P]ersons give meaning to their lives and relationships by storying their experience.... [I]n interacting with others in the performance of these stories, they are active in the shaping of their lives and relationships."[9] White argues that many people come to a therapist or psychiatrist because they are

> situated in stories that others have about him...and...these stories...allow insufficient space for the performance of the person's preferred stories.... Or the person is actively participating in the performance of stories that she finds unhelpful, unsatisfying, and dead-ended, and...these stories do not sufficiently encapsulate the person's lived experience or are very significantly contradicted by important aspects of the person's lived experience. (P. 14)

Psychiatrist Bradley Lewis has discussed the problem of a psychiatry that continues to behave as a modernist project with the goals and beliefs of the Enlightenment.[10] Lewis argues that psychiatry and patients would be better served if the theories, knowledge, and values of the postmodern perspective were embraced. He envisions a postmodern psychiatry in which the current quest for objective truth is transformed. Professionals join their patient's struggle in the search for what is most beneficial. Meaning-making is elevated and given a status equal to those of problem-solving and diagnosing. Faith in categories and methods are challenged by postmodern skepticism toward grand truths. Humility and tolerance of uncertainty are made acceptable in the patient-professional relationship. The goal-directed activities of progress and improvement are modified by the values of struggle and compromise. Personal responsibility is supported and encouraged.

Narrative can anchor psychiatry and the other behavioral health disciplines in the humility and compassion that can best serve patients in their suffering and can provide much-needed resistance to the current financial and cultural forces that are trampling on the needs of individuals with mental suffering. Narrative encourages practitioners of the behavioral health disciplines to envision and direct themselves toward worthy goals and purposes now eclipsed by the relentless biological reductionism that holds sway in contemporary psychiatry: to recognize mental anguish and suffering, to understand the root complexities and causes of such suffering, to provide compassionate interventions anchored in practices of informed consent and respect for persons, to participate with and join patients in meaning-making activity, and to not only treat and remove symptoms but to ameliorate suffering and pain whenever possible.

Narrative offers psychiatrists and other behavioral health professionals additional benefits: "diseases" are understood as "illness experiences"; local understanding and individual solutions replace the one-category-and-one-treatment-strategy-fits-all mentality that is emerging in current treatment guideline protocols; diagnoses are understood as signifiers of great complexity rather than as solutions to clinical puzzles; pathology and symptoms are appreciated as elements of an individual person's suffering rather than as information to support biological and psychodynamic theories; persons are perceived as individuals rather than stereotyped as diagnostic entities; objectification of persons is replaced with the process of intersubjective discovery through conversation and dialogue; and the tragic trend toward the commodification of persons and their symptoms is resisted through a return to professional integrity and humility that refuses to oversimplify and inadequately respond to the suffering of the patient. Professional responsibility cannot be ignored if one is no longer coopted by the economic and political forces that oversimplify and inadequately understand the needs of those with mental anguish.

In this chapter, the psychodynamic and biologic perspectives embedded in the biopsychosocial model in psychiatry and behavioral health are presented as inadequate to address the current crisis in psychiatric and behavioral health care. Narrative theories and methods offer a unique and fresh way of viewing the patient-professional relationship and the goals of that relationship in the practice of psychiatry and other behavioral health disciplines. Clinical and ethical decision-making in the patient-professional relationship are made more robust through narrative methods and understanding.

NOTES

1. The terms *psychiatry* and *psychotherapy* will be used in this chapter. I intend that the reader consider other behavioral health practices as well.
2. Although some might argue that some of the behavioral health fields are not "of medicine," the current reimbursement reality in U.S. health care reinforces the connection

between medicine and all of the behavioral health fields. Therefore, many of the ethical issues relevant to medicine are also important to the behavioral health fields, including psychiatry.

3. George Engel, "The Need for a New Medical Model: A Challenge for Biomedicine," *Science* 196 (1977): 129–36.

4. See Daniel Callahan, "The Goals of Medicine: Setting New Priorities," *Hastings Center Report* (November–December, 1996): S1–27.

5. Jacob A. Arlow, "Psychoanalysis," in *Current Psychotherapies*, ed. Raymond J. Corsini and Danny Wedding, 4th ed. (Itasca, IL: Peacock, 1989), 19–62.

6. T. M. Luhrmann, *Of Two Minds: The Growing Disorder in American Psychiatry* (New York: Alfred A. Knopf, 2000), 6.

7. David B. Morris, *Illness and Culture in the Postmodern Age* (Berkeley: University of California Press, 1998), 73.

8. Arthur Kleinman, *The Illness Narratives: Suffering, Healing, and the Human Condition* (New York: Basic Books, 1988), 50.

9. Michael White and David Epston, *Narrative Means to Therapeutic Ends* (New York: W. W. Norton, 1990), 13. Subsequent page references to this work appear in parentheses in the text.

10. Bradley Lewis, "Psychiatry and Postmodern Theory," *Journal of Medical Humanities* 21, no. 2 (2000): 71–84.

CHAPTER 14

IN THE ABSENCE OF NARRATIVE
JULIA E. CONNELLY

THE EVERYDAY LIFE

P rimary care medicine is concerned with everyday life. Here, ethical dilemmas arise from the lived life—individual preferences, beliefs, attitudes, choices, and decisions, and how individuals interact with one another as well as care for one another.[1] Ethical dilemmas in primary care are often subtle, but they are not invisible; most are recognized easily by careful observers. These dilemmas are no less important to the individuals involved than are the dramatic conundrums that touch the lives of hospitalized persons. For instance, an office patient with active gastrointestinal bleeding who refuses hospitalization despite a hematocrit of twenty may die at home due to further bleeding. The ethical dilemmas of primary care are different from those occurring in the hospital setting, but they are no less meaningful.

ON PRESENTING CASES

Narrative informs clinical medicine. Understanding such narrative works as pathographies, novels of illness and healing, and memoirs about medical practice enhances personal awareness, expands the physician's concept of the patient's illness experience, enables interpersonal connections and recognition of emotions, and thereby offers a fuller understanding of the moral life as enacted in health care.[2]

Patients' stories as heard and then interpreted by physicians are narratives too. Such clinical cases can, like literature, demonstrate particular points about the moral life. The retelling of these stories by physicians, nurses, or members of the ethics team is also a narrative activity. Such retelling may have consequences for the listeners, just as reading a poem may influence the reader in some deep way.[3] And the decision to retell a specific story is likely to be motivated by personal reasons of the teller, such as the wish to help the patient, to ensure proper care, to clarify or understand some aspect of the physician's life, or to bear witness in some way with the person who is suffering. Tod Chambers suggests that the reasons the teller "tells" need to be shared with the listeners of the case.[4]

The case I will present from my clinical practice is not unusual, but it stands out because it illuminates several points about narrative. I have chosen it for several reasons. First, many opportunities are present in clinical practice to ignore or overlook the patient's narrative. When the physician is too busy to listen or feel, too distracted to recognize the patient's need to engage in conversation, or underprepared in the skills of communication and psychological understanding, the patient may not be allowed or encouraged to tell his or her story.[5] In the absence of the patient's narrative, medical care fails *and is unethical,* a point I will demonstrate through the case.

Second, the case illustrates the essential nature of narrative in bioethics as well as the limitations of bioethical principlism when applied in isolation. Using the principles of bioethics in the clinical setting provides a framework for reflection, enhances the physician's understanding of the conflicts present in the moment, and clarifies the source of some of the social and psychological aspects of the interaction.[6] Without knowledge of the principles, the physician may not recognize ethical dilemmas or accurately categorize particular happenings. However, much more is needed in order to provide understanding and personal meaning. Knowledge of the principles is not enough.[7]

Narrative knowledge—comprehension of the specific, unique, detailed, and situated individual story—is needed to guide the relational aspects of care and the choices and decisions that often follow.[8] The actual narrative work of recognizing, absorbing, reflecting upon, and coming to at least provisional conclusions about the meaning of what the patient says and what to do about it is accomplished while talking with the patient, doing the physical examination, making diagnostic and therapeutic decisions, and writing prescriptions. All of it occurs seemingly at once in the rush and blur of practice. And after all is said and done in the patient's presence, the physician is left alone to interpret and evaluate his or her clinical and ethical actions. With whatever help is available from abstract principles and in view of whatever occurs between the doctor and the patient, the physician must rigorously examine and critique his or her interior processes—those events that occur deep down within the person of the physician. Even if, as suggested by Kate Scannell, the physician's aim is to be a "good" doctor, he or she has little guidance about how to achieve that aim.[9] Although the doctor may have the personal and professional commitment to uphold the ethical principle of beneficence, how is the upholding to be judged? Who decides on the quality and character of the physician's actions; who can tell whether or not this or that specific action is beneficent? Who is the judge?

In the office practice of primary care, the physician is left to be his or her own judge, deciding in seclusion if he or she is a "good" doctor. The physician's assessments of self—of whether his or her actions are beneficent or ethical—may or may not be accurate. A process of care based solely on principles of bioethics is risky if the physician is the sole evaluator of his or her actions. The principlist approach does not acknowledge the need for and the extreme difficulty of such ongoing internal assessment. So the principles have to be accompanied by methods or practices that support further understandings of the individual patient, the individual physician, and the therapeutic relationship as it evolves. The case I present addresses my interests in the areas of self-awareness, reflection, or self-knowledge, including potential revelations and inherent limitations of practices devoted to these goals. I aim to show that understanding through narrative may shed light on such critical yet subtle aspects of ethical practice.

Finally, the third reason for presenting this case is that many aspects of the case touched me. The whole story is a treasure; I want to remember it, and telling it ensures this.

THE CASE: WHEN THE PATIENT'S MIND IS SEVERELY LIMITED

One of my longtime patients, Emma, now seventy-five years old, called recently. She asked me, "Will you take on my brother?" Confused for the past year, he had managed to get by, but now he is in a crisis. A year ago, his physician diagnosed Alzheimer's disease, but "he wouldn't listen" to her.

Recently I have been thinking about patients with Alzheimer's disease. In fact, the voice of Cary Henderson, professor of history at James Madison University, still reverberates in my brain: his tone husky yet delicate and sweet, his cadence halting as he searched for long-lost nouns. Diagnosed with Alzheimer's disease at the age of fifty-six when a brain biopsy unexpectedly revealed the disease, he now lives in a nursing home and is unable to communicate. However, his ruminations and confabulations as well as his occasionally successful attempts to share and explain his life with Alzheimer's disease have been preserved on tape from the days he dictated his thoughts to himself. His wife Ruth, his daughter Jackie, and *Washington Post* photographer Nancy Andrews published *Partial View: An Alzheimer's Journal*, which, photographically and in his words, provides a poignant, painful, and remarkable personal reflection on this illness.[10] During a recent conference at the University of Virginia, his tapes were played as Nancy Andrews showed her heart-stopping photographs of him—around the house, brushing his teeth, enjoying time with his family at Christmas, trying to negotiate a staircase—during his illness. His descriptions are uncanny. As I thought about "taking on" Emma's brother, I could hear Cary Henderson's voice in the recording:

> I would love to see some people with Alzheimer's not trying to stay in the shadows all the time but to say, damn it, we're people too. And we want to be talked to and respected as if we were honest to God real people. (P. 7)

A week later as I entered the exam room to see Emma's brother Andrew for the first time, I remembered Cary Henderson's request. Seated on the examination table, Andrew watched me carefully while tapping his fingers on the elbows of his crossed arms. He was a large man, probably six feet, three inches tall, and appeared to be about seventy years old. I introduced myself, visited a moment with his sister, then asked him, "How are you?"

I wanted to observe him: What trouble did he have expressing himself or finding the correct words? How well did he process his thoughts and convey his ideas? How did he respond emotionally? Did he recognize his own confusion if, in fact, he was confused?

> People with Alzheimer's do actually think—they may not think the same sort of things that normal people think, but they do think. They wonder how things happen, why things happen the way they are, and it's a mystery. (P. 21)

Within a few minutes, I knew because of his anomia and confabulations that he had Alzheimer's disease. And at that moment in the interview, I was face-to-face with my customary response when the patient's mind is severely limited—I wanted to turn away from Andrew and ask his sister to fill in the blanks for me: How long has Andrew had problems? Tell me about his life. What is his living situation and how is he doing with his daily activities? Is he driving? Can he prepare food? Who takes care of his finances? Has he talked about moving where he can get more care? What other difficulties are arising?

I wanted to be a "good" doctor, and I did not want to embarrass Andrew or hurt him by asking simple questions impossible for him to answer. Cary Henderson acknowledged being embarrassed, feeling ashamed when he forgot something:

> Being dense is a very big part of Alzheimer's....When I make a real blunder, I tend to get defensive about it, a sense of shame for not knowing what I should have known. And for not being able to think things and see things that I saw several years ago when I was a normal person, but everybody by this time knows I'm not a normal person— and I'm quite aware of that. (P. 36)

Also, I was pressed for time. A discussion with him, I feared, would take forever, yet I still would need to verify what he said, so I might as well ask his sister. My own denial, too, pushed me away from him. I didn't really want to experience the depths of his dysfunction and feel the dreadful impact of these changes on him. Just as I turned to speak to Emma, I heard Cary Henderson repeat his undying wish for those with Alzheimer's disease: "And we want to be talked to and respected as if we were honest to God real people" (p. 7).

Cary Henderson made it plain that being ignored by his physician or anyone else was worse than feeling ashamed. Feeling ignored left him feeling disrespected, unacknowledged, misunderstood, and helpless. Because of Cary, I knew I could not ignore Andrew; I needed to talk with him to the extent that he was able. I had to know where he was in coming to grips with his illness. Did he realize his deficits? How did he feel when unable to remember? Was he aware that he was no longer a "normal" person? And he needed to know through my actions that I saw him as a person and respected him as such, normal or not. I knew I must listen to his halting and confused speech, no matter how difficult it was for me and how long it took. I must try to understand whatever he wanted or needed to tell me.

Our conversation was "communication by association." No longer could he recall names of cities, body parts, household articles, friends, or things common in all of our lives. Names that connect us with others, enable us to say what is on our mind, and give us freedom to come and go as we please were almost all gone. I knew he had been in the army, so I asked about his military service. He got excited and said, "We went on to...the really big one, spread out everywhere. You know the one." Assuming he referred to a city, I guessed Calcutta after his sister indicated he served in India. "Yes, yes that was it!" he exclaimed. And he went into a long discussion about the women of India "who did all of the work." He told me his unit flew across "the hump," referring to the Himalayas.

Later I asked him, "Do you have allergies to any medicines?" He said something like, "The green is everywhere. I sneeze, I sneeze from it." I assumed he was allergic to grass pollen but had no words, no names. Without words for runny nose, he made a blowing sound and spoke of sneezing and running. He pointed to the box of Kleenex and said, "I use those." He had no words for any of these objects, none of the usual connections from his previous life, the life before Alzheimer's disease.

It was a fill-in-the-blank situation as we tried to understand each other. When we finished, I told him I had some concerns about his memory, and he said, "Yes, yes!" He agreed to have some blood tests done and to return in a week. Standing at the door with his sister, he said, "Thanks. Thanks! I, I like you." One step at a time, I thought to myself as I took a deep breath.

A week later Andrew and his sister returned. The laboratory tests were normal. My aim was to talk with him about moving to a local adult-care facility where his sister had made arrangements for his admission, if he would go.

I asked him, "So how are you doing since our visit last week?"

He replied, "It's been terrible the last three days. I've been so afraid. The windows moving and the...He waved his arms over his head as he made swaying movements with his body.

I guessed, "The wind?" We had had a recent violent electrical storm with high wind.

He responded looking terrified, "Yes, yes. It's been terrible. I can't take it anymore."

Then he reached into his back pocket and pulled out an envelope as he said, "I brought this, if you want to see." And he handed me two small faded photographs, two by three inches, with tattered, brown edges. They were childhood photographs. As a child, two or three years old, dressed in a long white, wrinkled nightshirt and boots laced to the knees, he stood on the sidewalk in front of a large white frame house. In the other one, he had fallen down and sat on the sidewalk, laughing. As we looked together, Andrew said, "I'm on my butt!" and laughed.

Then Andrew took two folded, worn, yellowed papers from his billfold and gave them to me without comment. One paper, dated 1946, was his honorable discharge from the U.S. Army following World War II, and the other listed awards he had received while in duty, including a note of congratulations for winning the war. He again spoke about going over "the hump," then he was silent.

We sat quietly for a while. What should I say or do? I told him he had a disease that results in progressive memory loss. "This is the reason you have problems recalling names." I told him he would get worse and that he should move to a place where he could have assistance during the day. He listened and nodded his head. Finally he agreed to visit the nursing home, but he was not sure that he would stay there. I promised to visit him there if he needed me to. Okay, just one step at a time, I thought.

ONE PERSON'S STORY

The contribution of narrative, in this case *Partial View*, a visually expanded pathography that describes the chilling existence of a person with Alzheimer's disease, informed my medical practice as no medical documentation of the disease has. In fact, medicine's scientific arm rarely looks into personal meaning or the felt experience of illness. The literary treatment not only offers questions for ethical reflection but also provides answers and guidance in clinical practice.[11] What, for instance, is life with Alzheimer's disease really like? Who are the individuals as human beings? What do they understand about their lives? How does it feel to have Alzheimer's, especially in its initial phases, when self-awareness remains? What relationships or personal connections are possible?

Partial View offers a perspective on a mysterious disease and allows the mystery to unfold and reveal the Alzheimer's patient as a person. Not only do the human qualities of the affected individual persist, the self persists. For instance, the intense longing for human connection, whether in established relationships or during encounters with physicians, nurses, staff, and others similarly affected, is revealed by Cary Henderson. Also, the desire to be respected as a person no matter what the losses, no matter how "abnormal" one feels, remains. Because of *Partial View*, I heard much of Andrew's story and to my surprise engaged in a very special and personal interaction with him. I doubt that I will meet another person with Alzheimer's disease or someone with altered mental capacities due to a stroke or mental retardation and not recall the lessons I learned from Cary Henderson and Andrew.

NARRATIVE KNOWLEDGE

Narrative knowledge addresses the particulars of the case, attends to multiple perspectives, and depends on descriptions of a specific or situated context and personal details that define meaning. It allows many possibilities to be present at once and recognizes the emotional aspects of living one's life. Although narrative's focus is on the specific, it suggests that the case or story told holds universal truths.[12] For instance, does Cary Henderson's life—his sense of loneliness and isolation and his feelings of being belittled and disrespected—represent a universal experience among patients with Alzheimer's disease? Or is his experience a unique personal one? The answer is unknowable since a collective experience of individuals with this illness is not available. Yet to be ignored socially is never comfortable, so why assume a disease would change one's response? If I had turned to Emma with my questions, Andrew would have been voiceless. There would be an absence of his narrative account of his life and illness. I would know very little about him, and our relationship would be superficial at best. There would be no personal, human connection between us. The possibility that I might harm Andrew, not by embarrassing him, but by ignoring him, forced me to abandon my customary way of interacting with patients with this disease.

ANOTHER VIEW

The principle of beneficence in medicine requires of the physician a positive contribution to the welfare of the individual patient.[13] But who assesses the physician's actions and who determines which actions are beneficent? Physicians have the opportunity to review and reflect on their own actions. Such personal assessments may lead to such questions as: What am I doing? Why am I doing this? What is my aim? Why do I feel or respond as I do? Despite self-reflection, physicians may still misunderstand or misinterpret some situations. Only after hearing Cary Henderson's voice and reading his narrative in *Partial View* did my perspective change regarding my customary interactional style with patients who are mentally impaired. Now I am aware that some individuals I have treated may have felt ignored and perhaps were left voiceless.

As I became fully aware that Andrew's mind was severely limited, several things happened to me. I slowly *became* his physician, and I became aware of my wish to protect him from even the harm that I might cause him in exposing the secret of his confusion. Cary Henderson's narrative weighed heavily on my experience, while slowly and steadily his words transformed me. Joanne Trautmann Banks has acknowledged this power of literature: "Narrative inevitably expresses and transforms who we are at every level of our being."[14] I was finding out in a very personal way that the narrative of one person, in this case Cary Henderson, can transform the experience of another, myself. Later I asked myself, "Why did I move away from Andrew? Why did I feel that I needed to protect him from my direct questions? Why was I concerned about embarrassing him?" Slowly, I began to realize that I was the one who might be embarrassed and that I was hiding behind my personal concerns. Andrew's loss is a horrible one, and it will continue until his total disconnection from the human race occurs. I did not have the capacity to be empathic with him.[15] I could not imagine his experience. Even to consider the possibility of losing my mind was too much. I did not want to enter the depths of this world of loss; the scientific aspects of plaques and tangles are painful enough. Talking with his sister would bypass his world and allow me to focus on the superficial aspects of his existence. I would be protected from the reality that he exists in this condition.

Instead, knowing at least some of Cary Henderson's narrative encouraged me to write Andrew's narrative as a way to help me face his losses. I asked Emma to read what I had written about her brother and for permission to publish it here. Emma as well as her daughter were grateful to have read what I wrote and granted me permission to publish this essay. At the time of writing, Andrew has agreed to move into the adult-care facility.

CONCLUSION

Narrative knowledge allows and encourages human connections. One shared story often triggers the telling of other stories by involved listeners, facilitates memories and personal reflections on past experiences, if only silently revealed, and creates an expanded awareness of the moment, including a recognition of the power of personal presence and connectedness. Narrative knowledge is acquired by careful attention to many levels of the interaction between the patient and the physician.[16] Many of the skills needed to acquire narrative knowledge are patient-centered interview techniques that encourage active listening,[17] understanding of the biopsychosocial model,[18] and careful reading and interpretation of the patient.[19] The physician must also struggle for a deep awareness and understanding of herself, both her personality and her true self. Here physicians need the capacity for being present with the patient, an understanding of their own personal intentions, beliefs, and values and the ability to set them aside in order to focus on the patient, the commitment to care for the patient as a person, and an acceptance of feelings as an integral aspect of patient care.[20] Such knowledge may be gained in solitude, but sharing one's experience through telling stories within a group (as in a Balint group) or reading narratives may further personal insights and improve the accuracy of self-reflection. To engage in practice designed to enhance self-knowledge is a commitment to improve health care. Without narrative, deep human contact is very difficult, especially in the setting of present-day medical practice.

NOTES

1. See Harmon L. Smith and Larry R. Churchill, *Professional Ethics and Primary Care Medicine* (Durham: Duke University Press, 1986); Robert Coles, "Medical Ethics and Living a Life," *New England Journal of Medicine* 301 (1979): 444–46; and Eric J. Cassell, *Doctoring: The Nature of Primary Care Medicine* (New York: Oxford University Press and the Milbank Memorial Fund, 1997), for examinations of primary care ethics.
2. See Rita Charon, Joanne Trautmann Banks, Julia E. Connelly, Anne Hunsaker Hawkins, Kathryn Montgomery (Hunter), Anne Hudson Jones, Martha Montello, and Suzanne Poirier, "Literature and Medicine: Contributions to Clinical Practice," *Annals*

of Internal Medicine 122 (1995): 599–606; Anne Hunsaker Hawkins, *Reconstructing Illness: Studies in Pathography,* 2nd ed. (West Lafayette, IN: Purdue University Press, 1999); and Arthur Frank, *At the Will of the Body: Reflections on Illness* (Boston: Houghton Mifflin, 1991), for studies of patients' and doctors' narratives of illness and how these texts help doctors in their practice.

3. Wayne Booth, "Literary Criticism and the Pursuit of Character," *Literature and Medicine* 20 (2001): 97–108. This essay is a transcript of a lecture delivered to the Society for Health and Human Values in Chicago, IL., November 1990.

4. Tod Chambers, *The Fiction of Bioethics: Cases as Literary Texts* (New York: Routledge, 1999).

5. See John L. Coulehan and Marian R. Block, *The Medical Interview* (Philadelphia: F. A. Davis Company, 1997); Eric J. Cassell, *Talking with Patients,* vol. 1, *The Theory of Doctor-Patient Communication* (Cambridge, MA: MIT Press, 1985); and Mack Lipkin, Samuel Putnam, and Aaron Lazare, eds., *The Medical Interview: Clinical Care, Education, and Research* (New York: Springer-Verlag, 1995), for the conceptual and practical foundations of medical interviewing skills.

6. Tom L. Beauchamp and James F. Childress, *Principles of Biomedical Ethics,* 4th ed. (New York: Oxford University Press, 1994).

7. Anne Hudson Jones, "Literature and Medicine: Narrative Ethics," *Lancet* 349 (1997): 1243–46.

8. See Kathryn Montgomery (Hunter), "Narrative," in *Encyclopedia of Bioethics,* ed. Warren T. Reich, rev. ed, vol. 4 (New York: Simon and Schuster Macmillan, 1995), 1789–94; and Trisha Greenhalgh and Brian Hurwitz, "Why Study Narrative?" in *Narrative Based Medicine: Dialogue and Discourse in Clinical Practice,* ed. Trisha Greenhalgh and Brian Hurwitz (London: BMJ Books, 1998), 3–16, for discussions of narrative's natural place in clinical practice.

9. Kate Scannell, *Death of the Good Doctor* (San Francisco: Cleis Press, 1999).

10. Cary Smith Henderson, Ruth D. Henderson, Jackie Henderson Main, and Nancy Andrews, *Partial View: An Alzheimer's Journal* (Dallas: Southern Methodist University Press, 1998). Page references to this work appear in parentheses in the text.

11. Julia E. Connelly, "The Whole Story: Tolstoy's 'The Death of Ivan Ilych' and Olsen's 'Tell Me a Riddle,'" *Literature and Medicine* 9 (1990): 150–61.

12. See Kathryn Montgomery (Hunter), *Doctors' Stories: Narrative Structure of Medical Knowledge* (Princeton: Princeton University Press, 1991); and Brian Hurwitz, "Narrative and the Practice of Medicine," *Lancet* 356 (2000): 2086–89.

13. Beauchamp and Childress, *Principles of Biomedical Ethics.*

14. Joanne Trautmann Banks, chapter 21 in this volume, 219).

15. Joanne Trautmann Banks, "Caring for People Who Cannot Respond," *Academic Medicine* 66 (1991): 202–3.

16. See Hurwitz, "Narrative"; and Montgomery (Hunter), *Doctors' Stories.*

17. See Cassell, *Talking with Patients*; and Coulehan and Block, *The Medical Interview.*

18. See Lipkin et al., *The Medical Interview.*

19. Rita Charon, "Doctor-Patient/Reader-Writer: Learning to Find the Text," *Soundings* 72 (1989): 137–52.

20. Julia E. Connelly, "Being in the Present Moment: Developing the Capacity for Mindfulness in Medicine," *Academic Medicine* 74 (1999): 420–24.

PART IV

CONSEQUENCES OF USING NARRATIVE METHODS

CHAPTER 15

NARRATIVE ETHICS AND INSTITUTIONAL IMPACT
HOWARD BRODY

What effect might a narrative "turn" in ethics have upon health care institutions? While much more work needs to be done to define "narrative ethics," I am interested in what Hilde Nelson has classified as telling, comparing, and invoking stories; that is, using narrative as part of moral reasoning, rather than merely as illustrative of moral conclusions derived from other methods of reasoning.[1] Arthur Frank has succinctly characterized narrative reasoning as thinking with stories rather than thinking about stories.[2] Regarding what narrative ethics is not, I shall adopt the blanket term *principlist* to refer to the most popular, non-narrative ways we have to approach medical-ethical decision-making today. Rita Charon, for one, has suggested that principlist and narrative ethics are ultimately complementary rather than competing.[3] I would prefer to keep open the prospect that principlist ethics will be shown someday to have irreducibly narrative roots. But we need not resolve this question here.

Narrative ethics may have a profound impact on health care institutions, making them much more democratic. To illustrate how this can be, I suggest that we focus on a case study reported recently by John Lantos, even though space prevents its being presented here with the degree of narrative depth and richness that this new way of approaching bioethics seems to demand:

> A 9-year-old girl has AIDS with chronic lung and kidney disease. She now requires total parenteral nutrition through a central line and will probably need dialysis within a year if she does not die sooner from other AIDS complications. The patient's mother also has AIDS and is likely to pre-decease the patient. The patient knows only that she has a chronic disease, and has wondered aloud if she has AIDS; her mother has told her "no." The mother has told the staff that she would like to tell her daughter the truth but has not done so because her own mother is adamant that the girl not be told. The patient is hospitalized in a large teaching hospital where the multiplicity of consultants and staff make it likely that someone will let the true diagnosis slip out. The physicians feel strongly that it is in the best interests of the child to be told the truth. The grandmother insists, "It is enough for the girl to know that she has kidney disease; why should you tell her that she is going to die [of AIDS]?"[4]

Principlist ethics originally set out to make all of society's institutions, including health care institutions, more democratic. Basic moral principles are supposed to be transparent even to those of minimal intelligence. To claim a place at the table where ethical issues are being discussed, the principlist alleges, all one has to do is to offer reasons for one's proposed course of action phrased in terms of these widely shared principles. There might be experts in the history and nature of moral philosophy, but there are no experts in making ethical decisions. No privileged elite can claim to own the process of deciding.

In practice, this is not quite the way it has gone. If it is a sign of democratization that patients' rights are taken much more seriously today in health care than they were several decades ago, then indeed principlism has had a stunning victory. But if nurses, allied health workers, and other hospital employees remain disempowered in the process, the victory is not as great as it seemed at first. One can still, today, go to a meeting of a hospital ethics committee and hear a lower-status allied health worker (usually female) make a statement that, if seriously considered, would cast doubts on the entire discussion up to that point—only to have the chair of the committee (usually male), after a momentary pause, proceed with the discussion as if nothing whatever had been said by anyone.[5]

One might attribute such a scene to the fact that the wrong people are on the committee, or that the chair lacks skills in group facilitation, but some of the problem lies with principlism itself. Principles turn out to be much less transparent than we first thought. In order to be most useful in conventional ethical decision-making processes, the principles have to be framed in quite an abstract and general way. That means that many blanks have to be filled in, often implicitly, when we come to "apply" the principles to any real-life decision. Principles tell us, for instance, to respect patients' autonomy, but what might it mean to respect the autonomy of Mr. Smith in room 1303? Principles cannot instruct us how to act unless we first add quite a long list of facts and assumptions about Mr. Smith, his mental capacity, how he relates to various people around him, his medical condition, and so forth. Some people with certain types of training—advanced training in moral philosophy or ethics or law—become very good, at least verbally, in making the jump from the abstract principles to the fleshed-out applications, even though at times verbal facility may actually hide some highly questionable assumptions. (Perhaps, in Mr. Smith's case, these persons present such a plausible argument that Mr. Smith is suffering from diminished mental capacity that we never realize how much this judgment reflects hidden biases about the cultural group to which Mr. Smith belongs.) Such professionals may come to be seen as the "ethics experts" whose word is taken very seriously by the institution, while the questions and concerns of those with less facility with the "game of principles" may be systematically discounted, particularly if those latter individuals occupy work roles that are already devalued.

The creation of an "ethics elite" could recur in narrative ethics if the day arrives when people come to earn degrees in or do fellowships in narrative ethics. But a major tenet of narrative ethics is that this must not occur. Telling stories is one of the first lessons preschool children learn; they quickly object if the impatient or sleepy parent starts to tell the story wrong, either in content or in form. Maybe an "ethics elite" can convince an ethics committee that they understand principles better than others, but it is going to be quite a bit harder to convince a committee that some members understand narratives better than others.

Principlist approaches can hide the questionable assumptions that occur in applying principles to real-life situations, and members of a powerful elite are privileged to make assumptions and never be questioned about them. Similarly, a powerful clique can grab the narrative podium and privilege its way of telling the story.[6] But a thorough understanding of narrative would not allow this to go unnoticed. Narrative, just like principles, requires the reader or listener to "fill in the blanks." However, no one ever hears a narrative told by another. Instead, we tell ourselves a "virtual narrative" based on the narrative we hear—perhaps closely based, perhaps only loosely based, depending both on the narrative and on ourselves.[7] When a significant character appears in the narrative—for example, "Grandmother"—there is seldom the time or space for the storyteller to exhaustively describe this particular version of "Grandmother," and so each listener fills in the gaps based on what he or she imagines grandmothers to be like. The "virtual narrative" told by a woman who was physically abused as a child by her grandmother will differ fundamentally from the "virtual narrative" told by a man whose grandmother was the only adult trying to protect him from the abuse of others. Once we grasp this point, it is harder to get away with a privileged interpretation of a narrative than with a privileged application of an ethical principle, because principles stand with one foot in a realm of theory and abstraction, while narratives stand with both feet upon the ground of earthy human experience, be it factual or fictional. While there is a good deal of theory about narratives, we do not need to appeal to that body of theory when doing narrative "work" in ethics; with principlism, however, the abstract dimension is unavoidable.

Let us assume that narrative structure and cohesion matter when doing bioethics. (Proof of this assumption emerges if one tries to give an ethics conference to hospital staff, using a "real" case study that "stops" prior to resolving the moral dilemma: the presenter will not get out of the room alive without telling the audience "what actually happened in the end.") Let us also imagine that ethics requires that not just any answer be right. Narratives must be criticized and tested; and as Booth claimed, the only definitive way to show that a narrative is false or misleading is to tell a better narrative.[8] That observation suggests that the work of the ethics committee would be that of trying to think of various ways to retell or reconstruct a narrative so that one sees new possibilities or realities not revealed by the first telling.[9]

Who is most likely to see a narrative in a new light and to be able to offer a creative and revelatory retelling? More often than not, it is a marginalized member of a group. For one thing, that member of the group is likely to be "different" from mainstream members to start with; else why be marginalized? For example, to stop seeing an ethics case the way the physicians see it and suddenly to see the case from the nurse's or the patient's family or the cleaning staff's point of view often provides the profound shift of perspective or "standpoint" that allows one to read a narrative in a fresh fashion and to acquire radically new ethical insights.

In his article based on the case of the young girl with AIDS, Lantos tries to give us various alternative readings in which the grandmother acts in the child's best interests by ensuring that the child does not learn of her diagnosis. Maybe Lantos's argument fails, and in the end it would be best for the child to be told, as carefully and as compassionately as possible. But no ethics committee deliberating this case ought to reach conclusions before those alternative narratives have been put out on the table for a full discussion. Which members would be best suited to do that? Probably those whose life experiences and perspectives were closest to that of the grandmother and her family would be best suited to offer those narrative reflections. And we could guess that those would not be the same individuals who would emerge as the "ethics elite" in a principlist approach.

If these reflections are valid or even plausible, then narrative ethics would eventually transform a health care institution in the direction of taking the ethical thoughts of the lower-echelon workers much more seriously than is currently the case. If we combine such a trend with another parallel development in institutional ethics—the claim that the ethics of the organization need attention from ethics committees just as do the ethics of clinical care—then we could see how the more democratic discussions that might occur within the ethics committee could have a far-reaching impact.[10]

One objection to this discussion might be that we have, once again, given narrative credit for doing what would have happened anyway had we simply resorted to a thoughtful application of principles. We tipped the scales by selecting for study a case that had very important cross-cultural elements. Good application of principles depends upon accurate knowledge of the facts of the case, and the patterns of behavior and belief within ethnic subcultures are sets of facts one must collect before making a final ethical decision. In the hospital cited by Lantos, the less powerful workers might be more likely than the ethics committee members to share an ethnic and cultural background with the grandmother. It is not surprising that they would therefore be able to provide important facts for the committee's deliberations. But it does not require a narrative approach to state the facts or to put the facts into the moral equation.

Objections to narrative ethics often take this general form. One reply, in this case, is to go back to the idea of the virtual narrative. What that insight reveals is that there is no such thing in ethics as a case that is not in some way a cross-cultural exercise: the teller of a story always speaks to the listener across a cultural gap of one sort or another. Perhaps I grew up in the same neighborhood as you did, and we went to the same school and the same church, and my grandparents or parents emigrated from the same country that yours emigrated from; that does not mean that I grew up inside your consciousness. I will always fill in the blanks of a narrative somewhat differently from the way you do. Either we will recognize this fact and lay our narrative interpretations out on the table side by side for comparison, or we will ignore this difference and lose something important from ethical discourse. Whether we call what is missing "just the facts" or narrative plenitude hardly matters.

I contend, therefore, that narrative approaches to bioethics have the potential to emphasize democratic processes within health care institutions. We had at first hoped that principlist ethics would accomplish this task, but principlism has, in practice, proved itself disappointing in this regard. Learning to hear the voices of those reluctant to speak up, or who tend to be discounted when they do speak up, is one of the most vital but currently underappreciated tasks in health care ethics today.

NOTES

1. Hilde Lindemann Nelson, "How to Do Things with Stories," in *Stories and Their Limits: Narrative Approaches to Bioethics*, ed. Hilde Lindemann Nelson (New York: Routledge, 1997), vii–xx.
2. Arthur Frank, *The Wounded Storyteller: Body, Illness, and Ethics* (Chicago: University of Chicago Press, 1995), 158.
3. Rita Charon, "Narrative Contributions to Medical Ethics: Recognition, Formulation, Interpretation, and Validation in the Practice of Ethics," in *A Matter of Principles?: Ferment in American Bioethics*, ed. Edwin Dubose, Ronald Hamel, and Lawrence O'Connell (Valley Forge, PA: Trinity Press International, 1994), 260–83.
4. John Lantos, "Should We Always Tell Children the Truth?" *Perspectives in Biology and Medicine* 40 (1996): 78–92.
5. Susan Kelly, Patricia Marshall, Lee Sanders, Thomas Raffin, and Barbara Koenig, "Understanding the Practice of Ethics Consultation: Results of an Ethnographic Multi-Site Study," *Journal of Clinical Ethics* 8 (1997): 136–49; and Judith Andre, personal communication, 1998.
6. T. Hugh Crawford, "The Politics of Narrative Form," *Literature and Medicine* 11 (1992): 147–62.
7. Jerome Bruner, *Actual Minds, Possible Worlds* (Cambridge, MA: Harvard University Press, 1986).
8. Wayne Booth, *The Company We Keep: An Ethics of Fiction* (Berkeley: University of California Press, 1988).
9. Howard Brody, "Applied Ethics: Don't Change the Subject," in *Clinical Ethics: Theory and Practice*, ed. Barry Hoffmaster, Benjamin Freedman, and Gwen Fraser (Clifton, NJ: Humana Press, 1989), 183–200.
10. American Society of Bioethics and Humanities, *Task Force Report on Standards for Bioethics Consultation* (Glenview, IL: American Society of Bioethics and Humanities, 1998).

CHAPTER 16

RECONSIDERING ACTION: DAY-TO-DAY ETHICS IN THE WORK OF MEDICINE
JOHN D. LANTOS

Leon Kass recently expressed some doubts about whether bioethics, as a discipline, has changed the way American doctors practice medicine, think about healing, care for the sick and suffering, or act toward patients. Kass entitled his essay "Where's the Action?" thus challenging bioethicists to examine what they *do* professionally, how what they do changes what doctors do, and whether the activities of bioethics might not be marginal or irrelevant to the "real" action of medicine.

"In the practice of ethics today, ..." Kass wrote, "the action is mostly talk. . . . It seeks to analyze and clarify moral argumentation; to establish or criticize grounds for justifying our decisions; to lay down rules and guidelines, principles and procedures for addressing ethical dilemmas; and, in some cases, to construct comprehensive theories of conduct centering around fundamental norms, called autonomy or utility or duty or equality or benevolence."[1] There is nothing inherently wrong with this compulsive theorizing, he suggests, but there is nothing about it that inevitably or even plausibly leads to right action. Theory can become an end in itself. Kass goes on to ask rhetorically, "What is the connection between this practice of ethical discourse, now vigorously pursued by ethicists and their collaborators, and ethical practice, that is, the deeds of medical practitioners, hospital administrators, public health officials, and the countless citizens who have dealings with them?" And his implicit answer is, "Not much."

In thus examining the impact of bioethics upon medicine, Kass was not particularly interested in the sorts of actions that frequently are the focus of bioethical theory. He was not looking to see whether doctors were performing euthanasia, withdrawing mechanical ventilation from terminally ill patients, or meticulously seeking informed consent for tests and procedures. Instead, he was more interested in the everyday, lower-profile actions, those that do not flow from conscious theorizing but that are instead the result of embedded ethical presumptions reflected in the least deliberative of our actions.

In Kass's spirit of inquiry, we really learn about medical ethics by observing how doctors greet their patients, whether they make eye contact with them, and whether they refer to patients by their first names or by honorifics. We see ethical transgressions when doctors unwittingly embarrass or humiliate patients by, for example, talking about them to others in their presence as if they were not there. Although these everyday, unthinking actions form the substrate of day-to-day interactions between doctors and patients, it is unclear whether they are the proper concern of bioethics. Governed, apparently, more by simple rules and habits than by careful moral deliberation and ratiocination, these tiny actions might appear to belong more to the realm of etiquette than to that of ethics. Nevertheless, they do make up the moral climate within which larger bioethical dilemmas occur.

One way to conceptualize the distinctions among these different types of actions and the different views of morality that extend from their consideration is to distinguish between deliberative action and habitual action. Mainstream bioethics focuses primarily on deliberative actions. These are the actions that we take when we think about who we are and what we do. They are the products of our highest powers of reasoning. They lead to articles in scholarly journals, to presidential commissions, or to federal legislation. In contrast, habitual actions are the seemingly automatic things that we do "without thinking." Even so, the latter type of action reveals at least as much about our moral nature as the former and thus may properly be the concern of ethics. By telling us about who we are when we are *not* thinking about who we are, such habitual actions suggest that "[m]oral life here flows from character—ingrained, concrete, steady, like a second nature."[2]

One problem with recognizing habitual actions as moral actions is that such actions seem to be almost involuntary. A doctor who treats patients respectfully and empathically does not seem to be making moral choices or deliberative decisions. Despite a growing research scholarship demonstrating that health professionals can develop interpersonal and intersubjective capacities to reach and understand their patients, mainstream medicine (and perhaps mainstream bioethics also) persists in thinking of these personal skills as fortuitous gifts. If a doctor addresses her patients as Ms. or Mr. and if she attentively drapes patients during the physical examination so that they are not unduly exposed, is she manifesting an innate gentleness and kindness or is she performing actions that we should view and evaluate as morally salient?[3]

We can clarify these distinctions between deliberative and habitual actions and their status as moral deeds by turning for help to literary studies and qualitative psychology. Twentieth-century fiction and psychology have, among other things, redirected our attention from notions of action and character that might be called external to those that might be called internal. External actions are those that we can see. Internal actions, in contrast, are those that must be intuited or self-reported. Traces of internal actions may be seen or overheard in the flowing of a stream-of-consciousness monologue or in the disconcerting Faulknerian contradictions among multiple perspectives reporting on one action. Action in the twentieth-century novel is not necessarily what happens out there in the world. It can equally well be what happens internally; the mythic psychic struggles of

Freudian psychoanalysis or the rhythmic lyrical inner monologues of a novel by
Virginia Woolf or James Joyce both suggest a way of thinking about action that
might apply to a character who is not "doing" anything at all. Such narratives can
be tense with suspense and drama, though there is little "plot" and, in many cases,
nothing really "happens." Instead, such novels acknowledge the locus of many
important actions to be in the inner workings of the mind itself—its imaginings,
its utterances, its desires, and its thoughts—rather than in the realm of purposive
deeds. When we think, or dream, or fantasize, or philosophize, we are in the realm
of these internal actions. We understand that the use of the mind indeed constitutes action, however unruly or ungovernable by will, but the mind's experiments
cannot be seen or judged whereas those of the body are publicly observable and
therefore open to evaluation. Thus, the two realms invite quite different sorts of
moral accountability.

The sorts of narratives that provide the clinical cases for modern bioethics are
less concerned with the ways in which people think and feel than with what they
say or do. These cases are, if you will, patterned after pre-twentieth-century novels. We ethicists are more concerned with judging whether actions are permissible
or impermissible than with deciding which thoughts, feelings, or facial expressions are appropriate. We endorse a notion of autonomy in which the expressed
desires of competent individuals are privileged to an extraordinary degree (at least
those desires that govern choices about actions), while the thoughts or feelings
that underlie those expressions are thought to be either unknowable or irrelevant.
This approach entails a radically constricted, almost cartoonish notion of what it
means for someone to "do" something, just as it entails a notion of "autonomy"
that would be unrecognizable to Kant.

This approach, perhaps, is congruent with and reflects the nature of modern
medicine. Doctors today are action-oriented. Doctors do things. They question,
prod, and prescribe. They make an incision, insert a catheter, or ligate a vessel.
They are defined by and rewarded for these actions of intrusion or intervention.
In addition, of course, they take other actions. They sometimes ignore, misunderstand, or abandon. Sometimes they insult, offend, or injure. But the inner workings of the doctor's heart or mind, the flow of thoughts or feelings, the stream of
the doctor's consciousness, is not constitutive of a doctor's self-definition or, to a
great extent, to our social understanding of the important moral qualities that
make a doctor "good" or "bad."

In the world in which these doctors act, patients seem, by contrast, passive.
People generally become patients not when they do something but when something happens to them—they are hit by a bus, they develop cancer. Illness is composed of such involuntary actions as vomiting, swelling, coughing, and losing
function. This passivity is most striking in hospitalized patients, since they tend to
be the sickest, to be almost unimaginably sick in some cases, kept alive by the
sometimes miraculous, sometimes gruesome technology of the modern hospital.
During the illnesses of such patients, the action of health care remains more than
ever in the domain of the doctor. In fact, patients are "doing" a great deal by

enduring sickness, but their actions differ so fundamentally from the interventional or intrusive actions of doctors that they might not be recognized as actions at all.

The contrast between the interventional actions of doctors and the enduring actions of patients forms, to a large degree, the fundamental incompatibility and inharmoniousness upon which rest many of the troubles between doctors and patients. It is a glaring incompatibility, because, like in Faulkner's *The Sound and the Fury* or *As I Lay Dying*, the very nature of doctoring or being sick depends on the viewpoint from which it is observed. In stories that doctors tell about illness and healing (for example, Samuel Shem's *The House of God*,[4] Richard Selzer's *Mortal Lessons*,[5] David Hilfiker's *Healing the Wounds*,[6] and Perri Klass's *Other Women's Children*[7]), the doctors are essential, empathetic, engaged participants in the patients' stories (and, indeed, perhaps these particular doctor-writers are). In stark contrast, when patients or family members write of illness (and here, I'm thinking of such works as Philip Roth's *Patrimony*,[8] Evan Handler's *Time on Fire*,[9] Oliver Sacks's *A Leg to Stand On*,[10] and Arthur Frank's *At the Will of the Body*,[11]) the distant, unknowable, and unreachable doctors play small and almost inconsequential roles in the story that patients have to tell.

This incommensurability between being a patient and being a doctor renders the two viewpoints nearly unreconcilable. Nonetheless, much of modern bioethics seeks to alter this dichotomy by transforming patients into "active" participants in their care. Patients are conceptualized by a roll-up-your-sleeves bioethics as autonomous, as sharing in the decision-making, as active consumers of health care. They shop, compare, choose, and consume. Some patients can play this role, but they are, for the most part, the healthy patients. The sicker the patient, the less active they can be in this sense, and the less able they are to play the role demanded of them by this gesture of bioethics.

Again, the practice and theory of twentieth-century literature can help us in making sense of these dichotomies. Joyce, Woolf, Faulkner, and T. S. Eliot chose to look beyond the hero of the eighteenth-century picaresque novel or the hero of the nineteenth-century realist novel, heroes like Robinson Crusoe or David Copperfield who *did* things in the external world that declared their beliefs and character. Twentieth-century writers replaced these kinds of heroes with heroes like Mrs. Dalloway and Stephen Dedalus, heroes whose reflective consciousness and inner lives supplied the novel's action. Perhaps we can think of the impasse within contemporary medicine in these literary terms. Doctors' interventional or intrusive actions align them with eighteenth and nineteenth-century heroes who impress themselves on the external world through deeds and derring-do. Patients' endurance and ungovernable movements of mind and body align them with the reflective heroes of twentieth-century novels. To ask, as mainstream bioethics does, that patients relinquish their "twentieth-century" preoccupations to try to become, like their doctors, active in derring-do might be short-sighted or even regressive. Rather than valorizing the kinds of actions that doctors are good at, perhaps bioethicists might want to examine with more respect those actions that patients perform—those reflective, twentieth-century actions of brooding and giving oneself over to the ungovernable. And with the help of Woolf and Joyce, we also see now that those habitual actions of doctors—acts that emanate from ingrained habit or innate kindness—might also constitute this twentieth-century type of action that proceeds not from acts of will but from moments of being. We might be able to reconcile doctors' perspectives or behaviors with patients' perspectives or behaviors if we concentrate not on the deliberative actions of doctors but on their habitual actions.

At its best, ethics calls attention to moral problems that might go unnoticed. Like psychologists, novelists of the early twentieth century often paid attention to microscopic areas of moral deliberation—the moment between a thought and its suppression or the hesitation that might precede a question about a delicate topic. These unseen actions of the inner life might be the areas that reveal truths about our essential makeup. By focusing on these nontraditional notions of moral action, we bioethicists might be able to transcend shallow obsessions with the thin layer of our mind that directs conscious and deliberative action.

In avoiding the messy areas of consciousness and habits of being in favor of more finite and definable problems, bioethics seems as rooted in a pre-twentieth-century notion of knowledge and being as is biomedicine, which, for all its fancy science, is stuck in a nineteenth-century positivistic epistemology. Both bioethics and medicine imagine that truths are "out there" somewhere, to be directly observed and definitively characterized. However, since the twentieth century, both literature and the philosophy of science have become increasingly concerned with contingency, with the essential limits of the knowability of the world, and with the ineradicable link between tale and teller and between knowledge and knower. If brought into the clinical world, these insights might change the way we think of ethical relationships between doctors and patients.

These are not either/or distinctions. The world is big enough and manifold enough to hold Woolfian clinicians and Dickensian ethicists. But the shift that I am describing and advocating would allow both the clinician and the ethicist to at least recognize the existence of a world of moral deliberation that seems to have escaped critical scrutiny. It is the world in which the important question is not whether or not a DNR order is "permissible" in a particular case but what sort of conversation ought to take place before such an order is considered. It is a world in which the important question is not whether euthanasia should or should not be legalized but instead is how we can face our own mortality and the mortality of those we love, how we can care for those dying in pain without being overwhelmed by our own pain. It is a world in which actions and even words are seen as valuable in and of themselves, perhaps most valuable for what they suggest to us about inner life and inner moral struggles. Philosopher and psychoanalyst Jonathan Lear suggests that Freud is the modern philosopher most in tune with the implications of this sort of inquiry for both personal and political morality.[12] We can achieve neither accountability nor justice until we understand the springs of our identity and the motives of our actions.

It is surprisingly unfashionable in ethics to think about moral responsibility for things that we do not deliberate about or to think about actions that may seem automatic, everyday, picayune, or mundane. Habitual actions such as where we stand when we talk to a patient, whether we make eye contact, how long we pause to listen for answers to our questions, whether we allow ourselves to feel what the patient is feeling and to hear what the patient is saying contribute much of the meaning to doctors' behavior. Simultaneously, they are the actions that allow doctors to recognize who their patients are. By attending to such actions, doctors—and bioethicists—might be able to release themselves from their nineteenth-century derring-do of deliberative action to join their patients in enduring and reflecting on the habits of sickness and healing. Perhaps a narrative ethics can help them to do that. For these are precisely the actions that form the fabric of moral life, while the other, rarer and more deliberative actions form, at best, some of the patterns that are woven into that fabric. The complexity of our moral tapestries depends upon both.

NOTES

1. Leon Kass, "Practicing Ethics: Where Is the Action?" *Hastings Center Report* 20, no. 1 (1990): 6.
2. Ibid., 10.
3. Mack Lipkin, Samuel Putnam, and Aaron Lazare, eds., *The Medical Interview: Clinical Care, Education, and Research* (New York: Springer-Verlag, 1995).
4. Samuel Shem, *The House of God* (New York: Dell, 1978).
5. Richard Selzer, *Mortal Lessons* (San Diego: Harcourt, Brace, 1996).
6. David Hilfiker, *Healing the Wounds* (Omaha: Creighton University Press, 1998).
7. Perri Klass, *Other Women's Children* (New York: Random House, 1990).
8. Philip Roth, *Patrimony* (New York: Simon and Schuster, 1991).
9. Evan Handler, *Time on Fire: My Comedy of Terrors* (New York: Henry Holt, 1997).
10. Oliver Sacks, *A Leg to Stand On* (New York: Touchstone, 1998).
11. Arthur Frank, *At the Will of the Body: Reflections on Illness* (Boston: Houghton Mifflin, 1991).
12. Jonathan Lear, *Open Minded: Working out the Logic of the Soul* (Cambridge, MA: Harvard University Press, 1998).

CHAPTER 17

THE COLOR OF THE WALLPAPER: TRAINING FOR NARRATIVE ETHICS
ANNE HUDSON JONES

N arrative capacity seems to be an innate human ability.[1] However natural a part of the human equipment, narrative skill can be developed by exposure to environments rich in stories. Thus, even if people were all born with exactly the same narrative capacity, the narrative competence of adults would vary. Just as natural musical talent can be enhanced by the study and practice of music, narrative capacity can be enhanced by the study of literature and the interpretation of complex texts. One consequence of the increasing interest in narrative ethics is the need to think about the kind of training that can enhance the natural narrative capacities of those ethicists whose professional training has not been focused on the study of literature or narrative.

NARRATIVE COMPETENCE

Before good answers can be offered as to *how* such training can be provided, the more basic question must be answered: What are the narrative skills that help clinicians and ethicists carry out their work? Narrative competence for clinical and ethical work includes at least the following skills: first, the reading and interpreting of complex texts; second, the writing and oral telling of complex clinical and ethical texts; third, the interpersonal relational and empathic capacities that depend upon mastery of the first and second set of skills; and fourth, the ability to think with stories.

Reading and interpreting complex texts requires learning to ask and answer such questions as: Who is the narrator? Is the narrator reliable? From what perspective or point of view is the story told? What does this perspective leave out? Who are the other potential narrators of this story? What might their perspectives add? How can differences between narrators' stories be reconciled? What do individual readers bring to the story that influences their interpretations? How can differing interpretations be reconciled? If they can't be reconciled, how should a reader handle such ambiguity? What patterns emerge from the accumulating details, repetitions, images, and metaphors? That is, how does a skilled reader learn to recognize significant details that cohere in a pattern of meaning that makes sense of the whole? Knowing when the color of the wallpaper matters—and why—is the mark of a skilled reader and interpreter.[2] Interpretation is a skill that can be learned and practiced by reading complex texts with the guidance of highly skilled readers and interpreters.

The writing and oral telling of complex clinical and ethical texts are routinely required of clinicians and ethicists as they carry out their work. Whether they realize it or not, in writing or presenting cases, they make stylistic choices that influence the way their own stories will be read and interpreted.[3] Becoming aware of such stylistic choices and the effects these choices have on readers' or listeners' comprehension and interpretation—even on patients' compliance—is an important step in developing narrative competence.[4] Next comes learning to ask and answer such questions as: From what narrative stance should clinical or ethical events be described? Should this narrative stance change for different readers and audiences? How should awareness of the audience influence choices of diction, syntax, image, and metaphor? How does thinking in these terms help clinicians and ethicists become better writers and oral storytellers? And why does it matter?

Interpersonal relational and empathic capacities depend upon careful and respectful listening (reading, hearing, and interpreting the stories of patients, families, and others) and response (telling patients, family, and others clinical and ethical stories that are respectful and stylistically appropriate for differing levels of cognitive understanding and affective need). Mastery of the first two sets of narrative skills is necessary but not sufficient for mastery of this third level of narrative competence. Practiced at the highest level, narrative ethics as Arthur Kleinman and Arthur W. Frank have described it requires much more than skill at interviewing, taking a history, or even the empathic giving of bad news. It requires an existential *witnessing* of patients' suffering that goes beyond the often task-oriented medical encounter.[5] Kleinman, as physician, and Frank, as patient, both believe that clinicians should be willing to *be with* their patients in a human (as opposed to a professional) relationship that constitutes a more radical form of narrative ethics. Although this kind of witnessing may seem to go beyond basic narrative skills, it is an extension of respectful listening and is one of the consequential clinical dividends of narrative competence.

Thinking *with* stories, as conceptualized by Arthur W. Frank and David B. Morris, is a narratively complex skill relied upon by ethicists in making the singular and subtle distinctions of bioethics practice.[6] Such thinking uses the feelings and emotions inherent in stories as a complement or corrective to the prevailing biomedical ethics that attempts to rely solely on analytical reason. The power of stories to elicit sudden insight, or epiphany, and to motivate ethical action is well known, but it is also feared because stories have moved people to unethical action, as in, most famously, Nazi propaganda. A narrative ethics based on thinking with stories requires exploration of the complex relationship between emotion and reason in ethical thought and decision-making as well as in human behavior. It also requires careful reflection on what makes one story ethically "better" than another and experience in articulating how we know that.[7] In the clinical arena, it requires careful demonstration of how a narrative ethics approach to thinking about cases differs from an analytical ethics approach.

CONTRIBUTIONS OF LITERATURE AND MEDICINE

The current excitement and enthusiasm for narrative medicine and narrative ethics are the result of twenty-five years of work by literature and medical humanities scholars in clinics, hospitals, and schools of medicine, nursing, and allied health sciences throughout the United States and abroad.[8] Sometimes their work has been informal—directing elective reading groups or asking narrative questions while on rounds or in faculty and committee meetings. Other times their work has been structured formally into courses, seminars, or workshops. The cumulative effect of these many informal and formal efforts has been, first, to raise awareness of the importance of narrative in the work of medicine and of the necessity of knowing about narrative and stories in a more complete and effective bioethics for the future and, second, to develop consensus on the goals and methods of such pedagogy.

By now, many American medical and nursing schools have established elements of a curriculum in literature or narrative in medicine.[9] A goal of many such courses—to teach reading in the fullest sense—can be achieved only if students develop the interpretive skills that are also required in narrative ethics.[10] Medical students, nursing students, and residents in training—at least those in internal medicine, pediatrics, family medicine, and psychiatry—now have the opportunity or the requirement to develop skills in interpretation and the clinical imagination by writing about their clinical experiences in ordinary narrative language, reading accounts written by patients, doctors, and others about illness and doctoring, and receiving traditional literary training in the skills of close reading.[11] Rigorous study of the outcomes of such practices is under way and will be available to guide the development of such practices.

Despite the growth and popularity of literature-and-medicine courses during the past twenty-five years, many practicing clinicians and ethicists did not have the opportunity to take such courses during their professional training. Some of them might have received antinarrative training—that is to say, professional disciplinary training that dismisses as trivial or denounces as dangerous the skills and practices of the narrativist. Whether additive or recuperative, what kind of training can help ethicists and ethicists-in-training to develop narrative competence? Fortunately, there are many answers to this question. Some training methods are already available at many medical centers in the United States, and some fruitful future directions in training for narrative ethics can be considered.

CURRENT TRAINING PROGRAMS IN NARRATIVE MEDICINE
AND NARRATIVE ETHICS

The first step in accomplishing many of the activities described below is to identify colleagues in one's university's English or comparative literature department with an interest in medicine or illness. Many of the current concerns within literary studies—absence and mourning, testimony, intersubjectivity, liminality, contagion, reproduction—are enacted every day in clinics and hospitals, and many literary scholars and narratologists are eager to teach literature in a medical setting. Many medical centers have, with the collaboration of literary colleagues, offered some of the following training opportunities in narrative.

READING GROUPS

One simple and effective training method in narrative skills is a regularly scheduled reading group, guided by a teacher trained in literary studies. Because narrative insights depend on the transparency of thoughts to language, trainees have not only to read but also to talk about what they read, thereby enacting and confronting the multiplicity and contradiction among interpretations of good will and serious thought. The goals of such groups are not for students to master particular schools of critical theory but rather for them to grow in their ability to enter into, recognize, respect, and interpret the narrative worlds of others.

GRADUATE SEMINARS IN LITERARY STUDIES

Although not every bioethicist needs an M.A. or a Ph.D. in English, every literature department offers seminars that could be of great interest and utility to the bioethicist-in-training. One dividend of developing a relationship with one's local English department is that health professionals will be welcomed into undergraduate or graduate seminars on such topics as narratology, memory and autobiography, or literature as testimony as well as seminars on particular authors or texts.

WRITING ABOUT PATIENTS

It is no longer rare for doctors or students to be asked to write in ordinary language about patients under their care. For example, the residency program in family medicine at Columbia University developed a narrative ethics curriculum in which members of clinical teams write about patients whose care is ethically challenging. By writing from different points of view about a particular patient and then reading what one another writes, the interns and residents discover fresh and useful ways to think and act. Such writing activity is provided in a growing number of medical schools and hospitals for medical students at all levels, house officers, fellows, and faculty members.

WORKSHOPS AT PROFESSIONAL MEETINGS

Narrative ethics workshops offered at annual meetings of professional organizations can provide short, intensive training in close readings of a few texts or guided narrative writing about patients. Such workshops have been taught at meetings of the former Society for Health and Human Values, the American Society for Hospice and Palliative Medicine, the Society for General Internal Medicine, the American College of Physicians, the Society for Teachers of Family Medicine, and the American Society for Bioethics and Humanities. Not a replacement for ongoing narrative study, these one-time workshops can demonstrate the utility of developing narrative skills and can motivate professionals to embark on more sustained narrative practice.

INTENSIVE SHORT COURSES

During the past decade, Hiram College, Case Western Reserve, and Northwestern University have developed intensive, weeklong courses in narrative ethics. The first intensive short course in narrative ethics was offered in August 1992 at Hiram College, Hiram, Ohio, under the auspices of the Center for Literature, Medicine, and the Health Professions and continues to be offered yearly. With an original faculty that included Warren T. Reich, Kathryn Montgomery, Howard Brody, Brian H. Childs, Carol Donley, Martin Kohn, Jan Marta, and Robert M. Nelson, the residential seminars have taught works of fiction and poetry from many periods, critical theory, and conceptual works in bioethics. Over the years, the seminars have also addressed basic skills in narrative competence and such particular aspects of clinical bioethics as objectivity and emotion, narratives at the end of life, and narrative and chronic illness.

In 1996, Case Western Reserve University Medical School sponsored a weeklong intensive seminar in narrative ethics, directed by Kathryn Montgomery, that served as a course in its master's program in bioethics. The seminar examined the narrative nature of bioethics cases, literary concepts of truth and verisimilitude, and the relationships between casuistry and narrative ethics. In 1997, Northwestern University Medical School sponsored an intensive weeklong seminar entitled "Case Narrative and the Construction of Objectivity," taught by Kathryn Montgomery, Tod Chambers, William J. Donnelly, and Suzanne Poirier. Drawing participants from all over the country, the seminar focused on the construction of clinical cases and the ethics of representation in writing them. That such seminars are successful and oversubscribed may encourage others to offer them in the future.

FELLOWSHIPS AND CERTIFICATE PROGRAMS

Advanced training in narrative ethics is offered to clinicians or ethicists in postgraduate fellowships at Northwestern University Medical School and the Visiting

Scholars Program at the Institute for the Medical Humanities at the University of Texas Medical Branch at Galveston. The Certificate Program in Bioethics and Humanities offered by New York University and the Albert Einstein College of Medicine intercalates narrative training, under Rita Charon's direction, into its yearlong intensive training program. Existing fellowships and master's programs in bioethics may consider incorporating narrative training into their ethics programs.

TRAINING MODELS FOR THE FUTURE

ORIENTATION SESSIONS AND WORKSHOPS FOR ETHICS COMMITTEES

A series of seminars on narrative ethics could be offered at regular meetings of the hospital ethics committee to provide training in narrative competence. Such a seminar series might be developed by some with expertise in narrative ethics and offered regularly in different locations around the country, following the established model of IRB workshops sponsored by the Hastings Center. In the meantime, adding a session on narrative ethics to weekend courses for ethics committee members such as those offered by the Kennedy Institute of Ethics would seem a modest way to begin.

NARRATIVE CURRICULUM IN BIOETHICS TRAINING PROGRAMS

Currently available training programs in bioethics—including master's programs, certificate programs, and intensive summer seminars—may consider enlarging their offerings to include training in narrative skills. Such skills as close reading of literary and clinical texts, studying narrative theory salient to ethics consultation, and identifying reader response should become a uniform aspect of training for bioethics practice.

NATIONAL INSTITUTE FOR NARRATIVE IN MEDICINE

A national institute could serve as a clearinghouse for information and syllabi and could provide or identify funding to support workshops in narrative, regional summer short courses in narrative, and fellowships for the study of narrative in medicine. A national institute could also sponsor annual conferences where research about narrative medicine and narrative ethics could be presented.

INTERNATIONAL AFFILIATES

Interest in narrative-based medicine and narrative ethics is not confined to the United States. Fascinating work on narrative medicine is being done in the United Kingdom, Canada, and Australia. A national institute for narrative in medicine in the United States could systematically establish and maintain relationships and affiliations with similar programs throughout the world.

CONFERENCES AND PUBLICATIONS

Conferences devoted to narrative medicine and narrative ethics will continue to be important venues for encouraging multidisciplinary research and discussion. Articles in ethics journals and medical journals and books about narrative medicine and narrative ethics are proliferating. A goal for the near future might be to produce a report on narrative competencies similar to the recently published report on core competencies for consultation in health care ethics.[12]

CODA

More and more clinicians and ethicists seek ways of developing the skills and competencies that will help prepare them for a "bioethics for the twenty-first century."[13] We need to build on these informal and formal training efforts to develop more extensive models for training that will enhance our skills and improve our lives both as practitioners and as patients. I look forward to a future in which narrative methods and practices are a regular component of all training programs for bioethicists and clinicians.

NOTES

1. See the interview with Jerome Bruner, chapter 1 in this volume.
2. Anne Hudson Jones, "Darren's Case: Narrative Ethics in Perri Klass's *Other Women's Children*," *Journal of Medicine and Philosophy* 21, no. 3 (1996): 267–86; and K. Danner Clouser, "Philosophy, Literature, and Ethics: Let the Engagement Begin," *Journal of Medicine and Philosophy* 21, no. 3 (1996): 321–40.
3. Rita Charon, "Narrative Contributions to Medical Ethics: Recognition, Formulation, Interpretation, and Validation in the Practice of the Ethicist," in *A Matter of Principles? Ferment in U.S. Bioethics*, ed. Edwin R. Dubose, Ron P. Hamel, and Lawrence J. O'Connell (Valley Forge, PA: Trinity Press International, 1994), 260–83; and Tod S. Chambers, "The Bioethicist as Author: The Medical Ethics Case as Rhetorical Device," *Literature and Medicine* 13 (1994): 60–78.
4. Howard Brody, "My Story Is Broken; Can You Help Me Fix It?" *Literature and Medicine* 13 (1994): 79–92.
5. Arthur Kleinman, *The Illness Narratives: Suffering, Healing, and the Human Condition* (New York: Basic Books, 1988); and Arthur W. Frank, *The Wounded Storyteller: Body, Illness, and Ethics* (Chicago: University of Chicago Press, 1995).
6. See Frank, *The Wounded Storyteller*, 23–25, and David B. Morris, chapter 20 in this volume.
7. See Wayne C. Booth, chapter 2 in this volume.

8. Anne Hunsaker Hawkins and Marilyn Chandler McEntyre, eds., *Teaching Literature and Medicine* (New York: Modern Language Press, 2000).

9. Rita Charon, Joanne Trautmann Banks, Julia E. Connelly, Anne Hunsaker Hawkins, Kathryn Montgomery Hunter, Anne Hudson Jones, Martha Montello, and Suzanne Poirier, "Literature and Medicine: Contributions to Clinical Practice," *Annals of Internal Medicine* 122 (1995): 599–606; Kathryn Montgomery Hunter, Rita Charon, and John L. Coulehan, "The Study of Literature in Medical Education," *Academic Medicine* 70 (1995): 787–94; M. Faith McLellan and Anne Hudson Jones, "Why Literature and Medicine?" *Lancet* 348 (1996): 109–11; and Melinda Swenson and Sharon Sims, "Toward a Narrative-Centered Curriculum for Nurse Practitioners," *Journal of Nursing Education* 39 (2000): 109–15.

10. Joanne Trautmann, "The Wonders of Literature in Medical Education," in *The Role of the Humanities in Medical Education*, ed. Donnie J. Self (Norfolk, VA: Teagle and Little, 1978), 32–44.

11. Rita Charon, "Reading, Writing, and Doctoring: Literature and Medicine," *American Journal of the Medical Sciences* 319, no. 5 (2000): 285–91.

12. Society for Health and Human Values—Society for Bioethics Consultation Task Force on Standards for Bioethics Consultation, *Core Competencies for Health Care Ethics Consultation* (Glenview, IL: American Society for Bioethics and Humanities, 1998).

13. Jan Marta, "Toward a Bioethics for the Twenty-first Century: A Ricoeurian Poststructuralist Narrative Hermeneutic Approach to Informed Consent," in *Stories and Their Limits: Narrative Approaches to Bioethics*, ed. Hilde Lindemann Nelson (New York: Routledge, 1997), 198–212.

PART V

THE NARRATIVE FUTURE OF ETHICS PRACTICE

CHAPTER 18

THE HYPHENATED SPACE: LIMINALITY IN THE DOCTOR-PATIENT RELATIONSHIP
RONALD A. CARSON

The relationship of doctor to patient is primarily a moral, personal one.... Perhaps we should say that diagnosis and cure are processes which go on between doctor and patient.
          —Paul Ramsey *"Freedom and Responsibility in Medical and Sexual Ethics"*

Above all, physicians and patients must learn to converse with one another.
                    —Jay Katz, The Silent World of Doctor and Patient

The true locus of hermeneutics is this in-between.
                    —*Hans Georg Gadamer,* Truth and Method

I

T he hyphen is a key to understanding the relationship between patients and doctors. The hyphen simultaneously signifies separation and synergy, disjunction and conjunction. It calls attention to the distance between parties to the clinical encounter. And then, in the blink of an eye, it is a bridge across the divide.[1] The hyphen does double-duty. It signifies the reserve, the holding back, that is no doubt necessary when doctor and patient come together to consider matters personal and sometimes grave. And it reminds us that recasting one's life story in response to illness or injury is a joint venture requiring doctor and patient to work together to achieve what neither can accomplish individually.

Narrative theorists of medical ethics have put their minds to characterizing the many versions of the story-shaping conversation carried on in the liminal space, the in-between, of the doctor-patient relationship. Before selectively reviewing the work of some of these writers pertinent to my subject, and then articulating my own hermeneutic perspective, a few words about the context of narrative ethics may be apposite.

II

Nearly twenty years ago, Jay Katz provocatively proposed the metaphor of silence to characterize the world of doctor and patient. He argued that physicians' historical "caring but silent devotion to what they believed their patients' best interests dictated" had become tantamount to "psychological abandonment."[2] Moreover, Katz believed that, in modern medical practice, a patient's best interests could only be discovered in conversation with the patient. He understood conversation to be a necessary means toward shared decision-making, a model of the doctor-patient relationship grounded in the principle of self-determination that alone sustains the patient's integrity. He believed that clinical medicine was best served by a balance between the general principles of science and of ethics, on the one hand, and the particulars of each individual patient's care, on the other. Striking such a balance would occur in a silence-breaking dialogue between doctor and patient.

But as bioethics became professionalized in the early 1980s, the language of abstract principles gained hegemony over the particularistic idiom of conversation. Bioethicists became preoccupied with foundational concerns of applied philosophical ethics. Which ethical principles are most applicable in medicine, they asked, and how should those principles be prioritized when conflicts between them occur? Can patient autonomy be reconciled with physician beneficence? To address these foundational questions, mainstream bioethics availed itself of a contract view of the doctor-patient relationship. As medical knowledge had become more arcane and medical institutions more bureaucratic and crowded with apparatus and instrumentation, patients and doctors were at risk of becoming moral strangers to each other. In these circumstances the notion of contract was appealing in its implication that human relations are rooted in the uncoerced participation of free individuals. Historically, the idea of a social contract evolved as a challenge to the authoritarian power structures of church and state. Bioethics used this idea as an instrument of resistance against the modern aristocracy of biomedical science and technological medicine to effectively discredit medical paternalism and give pride of place to patient preference. But in so doing, it overlooked the fact that patients and doctors may not only have different preferences; they may experience the world differently. And, in assuming that social relations generally are motivated by self-interest, the notion of contract cannot sustain a relationship in which mutuality plays a significant part.

Narrative approaches aim to accommodate just this element of mutuality. Practitioners of narrative ethics share an attentiveness to the experiential dimensions of illness, a conviction that experiences of illness are story-shaped, and a commitment to relationality and reflexivity as preconditions for understanding such experiences. Beyond this shared attentiveness, conviction, and commitment, practitioners of narrative ethics theorize what transpires in interactions between patients and doctors variously.

III

Where there is friction in doctor-patient relations, Rita Charon perceives a clash of traditions. On the one side is medicine, with its case-historical method of determining how things always are beneath the symptoms that have surfaced. On the other side is the ailing person, with his or her sense of how it feels to be feeling poorly in just this way and no other, and for no apparent reason. The diagnostician deals in universals, the patient in particulars, and the two have trouble understanding each other. To bridge this gulf, Charon advocates the recovery and use of ordinary language by physicians, language that brings patient and doctor together in a relationship in which "subjective knowledge of the world (on the parts of both doctor and patient) matters as much as the objective gaze toward fixed norms."[3]

In her book *Doctors' Stories*, Kathryn Montgomery[4] argues that medicine is a narratively constructed body of practical knowledge and that the practice of medicine consists in adjusting this generalized abstract knowledge to individual cases of malady. The mechanism for making this adjustment is the case method.

The case, in Montgomery's view, is the basic unit of thought and discourse in medicine; it is a representational narrative, and it is "rigidly conventional."[5] Physicians are bound by communally established narrative forms that both guide the acquisition of medical knowledge and convey the physician's observations. Whether interviewing a patient or dictating a chart entry or consulting a colleague or presenting at rounds, physicians practice according to the discipline of the narrative conventions of the case method, taking prescribed steps from chief complaint through diagnosis to formulation of a plan of care. The doctor listens to the patient's version of events, transforms that story into a plausible medical plot, and returns the latter to the patient. The account a physician constructs aims to translate the patient's subjective experience into the recognizable discourse of medicine, to "represent" it in medical terms, to "objectify" it—which is to say, to figure out what it best matches when held to the template of traditional medical accounts of what counts as illness. The fundamental act of patient care consists in the construction of a metastory about the patient's story that makes sense of the events of illness by testing those events against "the taxonomy of diagnostic plots and settling on one that is sufficiently likely to warrant therapeutic intervention" (p. 129).

The success of a therapeutic intervention depends on the skillful return of the medical account of the patient's malady to the patient. For this, medical practitioners need "a narrative self-consciousness"; that is, "a recognition, first, that the patient is the source of narrative unsubsumed by the medical case and, second, that the case is a medical construct rather than a natural object" (p. 141). One can see how such self-consciousness might provide a hedge against crude reductions of the patient's experience, but it is not clear how doctors are to go about restoring the patient's medically replotted story to the patient, or how patients are to carry off such a complicated act of reappropriation. To the question of who gets to tell stories of sickness and how are they to be emplotted, Montgomery answers, "patients and doctors," in that order and according to the conventions of medical knowledge. The patient's story is experiential. The doctor takes in the patient's story, restructures it in medical terms, and returns it to the patient, saying, "This is what is going on beneath or behind your symptoms." The patient must then try to make sense of his or her illness in light of the abstractions of medical knowledge.

Montgomery acknowledges that the medical story is always secondary, derivative of the patient's account. Without the patient's story, the doctor would have nothing to work with. Montgomery is cognizant also of the danger that the medical representation of illness may reduce the illness to a disease without significant experiential remainder. The very purpose of the medical story is, after all, the identification and treatment of a disease. But in the absence of an account of the process by which the medical story is restored to the patient in a way that is meaningful in the context of the patient's life story, the medical story takes precedence. In the end it is the medical version of events that prevails, with all that that implies regarding the expropriation of the patient's experience.

Arthur Frank, too, observes that medicine's case method consigns medical professionals to thinking about patients' stories rather than with them. For Frank, "Thinking *with* stories is the basis of narrative ethics."[6] He develops a typology of illness narratives as "*listening devices*" to orient the ill person and those caring for him or her (p. 76). Although Frank acknowledges that medical decisions are likely to be more empathic when medical professionals invoke narrative knowledge, his interest in narrative has not been in the first instance as an aid to clinical decision-making. Instead, narrative knowledge enhances an ill person's ability to determine "*how to live a good life while being ill.*"[7] That said, in a recent exchange with Jeffrey Bishop, Frank has turned his attention more explicitly to the dialogical nature of narrative.[8]

Anne Hunsaker Hawkins's avowed aim in introducing the term *pathography* into medical ethics discourse is to distinguish (subjective, particularistic) biographical or autobiographical accounts of experiences of illness from medicine's (objective, universalistic) case-historical account. Then, having argued for the restoration of the patient's voice to the medical enterprise, she ends her study with a call for the voice of the physician to be heard as a counterpoint to patient pathographies. By this she means not reporting from a professional point of view but writing about what it is like to be a physician today, interacting with patients—the physician as person. "Only when we hear both the doctor's and the patient's voice will we have a medicine that is truly human."[9]

As literary approaches began to influence thinking about medical ethics in the late 1980s, writers of an interpretive bent, myself included,[10] drew heavily on the text analogy for understanding the doctor-patient relationship. I believe that the analogy remains promising,[11] but questions about what constitutes the text, and about how the reading gets done, and by whom, continue to be more complicated than we originally thought. In some early cautionary remarks on taking the text analogy too literally, Anne Hudson Jones wrote, "When the patient is capable of actively participating in constructing the narrative of his or her illness, the doctor should engage the patient in a process of collaborative interpretation and story construction.... Even when—or perhaps *especially* when—the patient is unable to participate fully in helping construct or correct the interpretations of his or her story, it is important to seek a dialogic reading."[12] In a later commentary on an article of mine on reflective practice, Jones saw more clearly than I at the time the pitfalls of thinking of the patient as text and the doctor as reader. Dialogical narrative ethics, she wrote, "presumes a nonhierarchical narrative paradigm,"[13] a point I now willingly concede, and to which I would add "and must strive to be radically egalitarian."

IV

As physicians and patients have attempted to break the silence noted by Katz two decades ago, they have often found themselves talking past each other. The narrative theorists of medical ethics to whose work I have made reference have identified a number of plausible reasons for this rift and have proposed a variety of remedies. They generally agree, however, that doctors and patients value experience differently. I believe that the relative paucity of meaningful conversation in the doctor-patient relationship is symptomatic of the continuing disappearance of narrative from the realm of living speech that Walter Benjamin noted in his reflections on storytelling in the 1930s. As "experience has fallen in value," Benjamin observed, our "ability to exchange experiences" is diminished, dependent as this ability most certainly is on narrative consciousness.[14] In other words, the ability to *relate* one's story depends on there being a *relationship* in which that story can be received, recognized, and responded to.

Narrative theorists of medical ethics are wagering that the fissures in the doctor-patient relationship can be healed by placing the patient's experience at the center of the clinical encounter and by animating dialogue about that experience. The dialogue will tack back and forth between the patient's story (What has brought the patient to the doctor just now, beyond the "chief complaint," and as a context for it?) and the doctor's ordinary sense of how things seem with the patient, impressions the doctor will check against the patient's experience. The doctor will certainly have recourse to the taxonomy of diagnostic plots in medicine's storehouse of practical wisdom, but that move will be secondary to the conversation and the interaction themselves, which will assume primary significance in a mutual search for understanding and for a livable future for the patient. Especially when dealing with chronic illness, this may seem more like muddling through together than the dispensing of expert advice, as is evident in this story told by Dr. David Hilfiker.[15]

It is Clint Wooder who serves Hilfiker communion on the Sunday morning at Christ House, a haven for homeless people, on which the story opens, a role reversal that makes sense only after the tale is told. Why Wooder is unabashedly beaming and Hilfiker is choked up becomes clear as the narrative unfolds. Participating together in the ritual of memory that is the Eucharist, Wooder gazes straight into the communicant's eyes, whereupon Hilfiker's vision is blurred by tears as he recalls his first encounter with Clint Wooder as a patient.

The doctor remembers being startled by the stark contrast between the patient's weathered face and hands and his pale, emaciated body, his belly bloated with fluid from years of heavy drinking. He also remembers Wooder's penetrating eyes, guileless and beckoning, eyes that trusted the doctor and took him in. Inexplicably, Wooder seemed to believe he had a future, although he lived close to the precipice of death and was convinced that he could not control his fatal urges. He was concerned about his health and kept his weekly appointments with Dr. Hilfiker. The doctor could do little more than monitor the patient's slow recovery from a recent drinking bout that had taken him to the very edge of the precipice. Wooder was now inching his way back from the edge by attending as many AA meetings as he could squeeze into a day and by otherwise making himself useful around the shelter. Hilfiker experienced both puzzlement and a curious kinship with this wreck of a man who continued to dream of carrying his own weight in the world, of having a place to call his own and the means to support himself.

After months of sobriety, Wooder grew agitated and threatening and implored Hilfiker to help him handle his conflicting urges to lash out at someone or to drown his rage in drink. Invested by now in Wooder's recovery and judging him to be psychologically stranded, Hilfiker set out on an arduous journey to get help. The obstacles were many, not all were surmountable, and the lessons to be learned were hard. Although Wooder had learned them long ago and continued nonetheless to dream of a way out, his would-be helper had to learn them all from scratch.

Hilfiker could find no therapist willing to take on a penniless, homeless man with a severe alcohol problem. He phoned friends, he followed leads, he turned up a sympathetic psychiatry resident who was, however, barely keeping up with patients who were worse off than Wooder. Meanwhile, Wooder was getting worse. When his rage made him momentarily unrecognizable to the doctor, Hilfiker decided to recommend hospitalization. Little did he know how empty was his offer. After a rollercoaster ride of a weekend, in and out of hospitals, voluntarily and involuntarily, Wooder was once again left to his own devices.

Against all expectations, Wooder remained sober and came back to the doctor for a few weeks. It is as if he was trying to give Hilfiker a chance to redeem himself from his ill-fated attempt at forced help. But trust had been compromised by Hilfiker's botched attempts to save Wooder from himself, and soon Clint was back on the streets and on the bottle. When next Hilfiker saw Wooder, he did not recognize him, so drunk and disheveled was he, his skin green, his eyes vacant.

His urge to rescue now subdued, his desire to help still strong, the doctor asked Wooder for permission to take him to the city's public detoxification unit. At first he refused, saying he was beyond help and that they, too, would turn him away. The doctor assured him that that would not happen and offered to accompany him. "I'll take you down. Will you let me take you to detox, Clint?" Wooder thought it over and then accepted. The doctor had one more hard lesson to learn, but he had redeemed himself with Wooder. Unbeknownst to Dr. Hilfiker, the two would again meet defeat on the next leg of their journey, but they would meet it together. Trust had been restored. It sustained them through their descent into the pit of a public hospital, the gates of which were guarded by a rule-bound lackey physician and a belligerent black attendant bent on driving home to this stuporous white hillbilly and this insistent white doctor how it feels to be marginal and powerless.

Desperate now, Hilfiker single-handedly undertook to dry Wooder out. When the attempt failed, as it was bound to, it left the two men angry, hopeless, and truly without options. Wooder returned to the streets to rein in his anger in the only way available to him. Hilfiker turned inward to grieve a double loss: the loss of his friend and the loss of innocence incurred by acknowledging his own professional limits. He now sadly recognized that some ends are beyond the reach of even the best will in the world.

With the passage of time, Hilfiker also came to understand that this trying experience with Clint Wooder had been a joint journey on which, instead of being Wooder's guide (as the doctor had naïvely thought of himself), it was Wooder who had taken Hilfiker along to learn a few of life's lessons. Hilfiker felt favored to have been singled out to learn firsthand about the vagaries of justice and mercy.

And about the unforcible intrusion of grace. Somehow, Wooder survived another bout with oblivion and returned to the shelter to begin yet again. The pattern of attempted recovery was familiar. Except this time, Wooder made it back far enough away from the edge of the precipice to get a part-time job, eventually a full-time job, and a small apartment of his own. The dreams he had once confided to the doctor were coming true, at least for the time being, which Hilfiker, well-taught, now knew is all the time any of us have.

So it is on the Sunday morning that frames this story that Hilfiker, awaiting his turn at the communion rail and trying to reflect on the meaning of the Eucharist, finds his attention focusing instead on Clint Wooder and the chalice in his hands. Wooder can barely contain his laughter as he repeats the ritual declaration, "This is the blood of Jesus." This is the wine, death-dealing when taken in solitude as an antidote to anger, transforming and life-giving when received in companionship to commemorate self-giving. As Hilfiker lifts the cup of kindness to his lips, his vision blurs with tears of gratitude. It is a moment of mutual recognition. The doctor is implicated. He has become a character in the patient's story. Moreover, in writing about Wooder and himself interacting, Hilfiker is present not only as doctor but also as narrator. As Hilfiker expresses Wooder's story, it becomes something new; it becomes Wooder's and Hilfiker's story in the telling.

V

I believe with Charles Taylor that "[w]e are, in a sense, surrounded by meaning."[16]
Contrasting representational (Enlightenment) and expressivist (Romantic) theories of meaning, Taylor identifies three key elements in the expressivist tradition.
We formulate matters of meaning in the activity of speaking. In so doing we bring
them more clearly to consciousness and, "in cases of genuine formulation, we only
know afterwards what we are trying to identify" (p. 258). In a way, the formative
becomes normative or, at the least, articulate where before it was inchoate.
Moreover, when we strike up a conversation about things that matter, what is
expected "is no longer just a matter for me, or for you, or for both of us severally,
but is now something for us, that is for us together" (p. 259).[17] The hyphen in the
doctor-patient relationship signifies common ground from which patient and
doctor can peruse the patient's experience together. Even when they misunderstand each other or are at odds, common ground is accessible to dialogical digging
beneath the surface of manifest differences. Perhaps "ground" is too static a
metaphor. Gadamer calls it simply "common experience," "a deep common
accord."[18] Elsewhere, Taylor draws on the metaphor of rhythm to help distinguish
coordinated monological action based on predictability of response (his example
is of running to a predetermined spot on a playing field where one knows another
is going to pass the ball) from open-ended dialogue. "Conversations with some
degree of ease and intimacy move beyond mere coordination and have a common
rhythm. The interlocutor not only listens but participates with head-nodding and
'unh-hunh' and the like, and at a certain point the 'semantic turn' passes over to
the other by common movement. The appropriate moment is felt by both partners together in virtue of the common rhythm."[19] Finally, following Taylor still, the
activity of engaging in conversation is not only expressive but constitutive as well.
Speaking and listening constitute our relationship, creating "the kinds of footings
we can be on with each other."[20] The in-between is established and shaped by what
I say to you, the way I behave toward you, by what you make of what I say and do,
and by how we both respond. Consider the following story, told by Terry Pringle.

Receiving the news of his son Eric's first relapse of leukemia, Terry Pringle
reflects, "As a child I always knew there were boundaries. A bully could chase me,
but would stop at the front door. My father might beat me, but would stop short
of killing me. We are subject to illness, but it can always be cured. We are safe
within these boundaries. And when I see the boundaries are imaginary, I feel
sick. . . . I want my son to live. I have never begged for anything in my adult life, but
now I am begging."[21]

Early in this moving narrative, Terry Pringle introduces readers to Dr. Pope,
the Abilene pediatrician who is to execute the medical decisions of the Houston
specialists responsible for treating Eric's leukemia. At first, Dr. Pope seems to
Brenda Pringle insufficiently concerned about her son. There are some miscom-
munications between Houston and Abilene regarding drug dosages, and it is

Eric's mother, not the doctors, who sorts things out. But Dr. Pope persists, staying in touch with Eric and his parents. "The words he speaks aren't nearly so important as the efforts he makes. We need at least one doctor to confirm that Eric is important to him, that he is thinking as well as acting, that he recognizes the treatment comes from a standardized schedule, but our son is not a compilation of statistics and probable responses" (p. 77).

The relationship between the child and the physician grows over time. Eric tells his parents that Dr. Pope is as skilled as the Houston specialists at doing a spinal tap. On another occasion, Eric objects to having to lie down to receive injections. "'Okay,' the doctor says, 'we'll do it your way'" (p. 136). Whenever there is a choice of physicians, Eric wants Dr. Pope.

As the Pringles begin to run out of medical options and decide to try an experimental drug, they call their pediatrician. "He asks Brenda how we are doing. 'Fine,' she said. 'Now tell me how you're really doing.' A friend tells us later that the doctor had asked him if anyone had heard from us; he had thought about us all day" (p. 96). When it becomes clear that cure will not come, Terry Pringle breaks down. "Once loosed, the sobs are unstoppable. I sit on the coffee table with my head in my hands; Dr. Pope crosses the room and pulls me up, embracing me. I understand instinctively the move he has made. We don't know each other well, he is as reserved as I am. And I know the steps across the room were long ones for him, not only to me, but out of a role that protects him. The doctor prays, 'Lord, this hurts'"(p. 136).

While the Pringles decide about next steps, the doctor listens. Do they want Eric hospitalized? No, they wish to keep him home. From then until the end, Dr. Pope attends Eric at home. When Eric's parents are overwhelmed by the burdens they bear, the doctor steps in, gently but steadily. It is a kind of sad, beautiful dance, with one partner leading for a time and then the other.

Terry Pringle telephones Dr. Pope in the middle of an October night to tell him that Eric has died. "He is there within a few minutes and sits beside Eric a long time, sniffing and rubbing Eric's arm and head. Before he checks for a heartbeat, he performs the same ritual he always has—rubbing and blowing on the stethoscope to warm it before touching it to Eric's chest" (p. 177).

In one of many valiant attempts to characterize *das Zwischenmenschliche* or *Zwischenmenschlichkeit*, the untranslatable German word that means a special something that happens between people when they are "in sync," taking each other seriously and holding each other in mutual regard, Martin Buber wrote, "In a real conversation ... what is essential does not take place in each of the participants or in a neutral world which includes the two and all other things; but it takes place between them in the most precise sense, as it were in a dimension which is accessible only to them."[22] As ethereal and mysterious as this may sound, what Buber had in mind is not something that happens only during the great thundering moments of life. This "connecting" also accompanies ordinary experiences and is often accompanied by a sense of surplus meaning—as when conversing with a sick child and his parents, and they with you, about how things are going and what to do next. And what are we to "do" with the surplus? Take note of it, take it in, reinvest it in the relationship, and pass it on.

VI

The ritual elements in the two stories I have retold bring me to some final thoughts about the liminality of the hyphenated space in the doctor-patient relationship. The concept of liminality (from the Latin *limen*, for "threshold"), coined by Arnold van Gennep and developed by Victor Turner[23] refers to the ritual "space" in which one is suspended, straddling or wavering between two worlds, neither here nor there, betwixt and between settled states of self, as in rites of passage or, by extension, when experiencing illness, especially life-threatening or self-threatening illness.

Liminal space is a place of ambiguity and anxiety, of no-longer and not-yet. To enter such a space is to slip one's moorings and be carried by currents toward one knows not where, to be in limbo. When illness threatens, we seek out experienced conversation partners, notably doctors, to help us get our bearings and get back on course. I want my doctor to tell me the medical meanings of my symptoms, to be sure, but I also want some help in grasping the personal significance of my malady. I want both to have my "otherness" acknowledged and to be recognized as still belonging to the tribe of the living. I want to understand what is happening to me, and for this I need to be understood. Hermeneutics reminds narrative ethics that understanding is fundamentally relational.[24]

David Hilfiker and Clint Wooder, and the Pringles and Dr. Pope, learned something they had not known, something that was unknowable, prior to their engaging each other in the liminal space of their respective relationships. They came to an understanding about the footings they could be on with each other. Beyond this new knowledge, they also acquired a richer sense of themselves as moral beings. By virtue of having been morally implicated in each other's lives, they were transformed, their spirits enlarged.

The hyphenated space in the doctor-patient relationship is a liminal place of ethical encounter, alternating voices and actions—back and forth, address and response—seeking mutually satisfactory meaning by means of which an illness that has threatened to fray or sever the storyline of a life can be woven into the fabric of that life. The hyphen points to the prospect of overcoming silence with meaningful conversation.

NOTES

1. Writing in a different context but somewhat analogously, Hans-Georg Gadamer avers, "[I]t seems to be generally characteristic for the emergence of the hermeneutical problem as such that a situation must exist where something remote has to be brought

nearer, a strangeness overcome, a bridge built between 'once' and 'now.'" "Rhetoric, Hermeneutics, and the Critique of Ideology: Metacritical Comments on *Truth and Method*," in *The Hermeneutics Reader*, ed. Kurt Mueller-Vollmer (New York: Continuum, 1988). Originally published in German in 1976.

2. Jay Katz, *The Silent World of Doctor and Patient* (New York: The Free Press, 1984), 207, 208. Subsequent page references to this work appear in parentheses in the text.

3. Rita Charon, "To Build a Case: Medical Histories as Traditions in Conflict," *Literature and Medicine* 11 (Spring 1992), 130. See also Charon's "Narrative Contributions to Medical Ethics: Recognition, Formulation, Interpretation, and Validation in the Practice of the Ethicist," in *A Matter of Principles? Ferment in U.S. Bioethics*, ed. Edwin R. Dubose, Ronald P. Hamel, and Laurence J. O'Connell (Valley Forge, PA: Trinity Press International, 1994), 260–83.

4. The author's name at the time of publication was Kathryn Montgomery Hunter.

5. Kathryn Montgomery Hunter, *Doctors' Stories: The Narrative Structure of Medical Knowledge* (Princeton: Princeton University Press, 1991), 54. Subsequent page references to this work appear in parentheses in the text.

6. Arthur W. Frank, *The Wounded Storyteller: Body, Illness, and Ethics* (Chicago: University of Chicago Press, 1995), 158. Subsequent page references to this work appear in parentheses in the text.

7. Ibid., 156. As recently as 1997, Frank wrote, "[M]y goal is restoring the patient's voice to the patients themselves or enhancing a developing self-consciousness among ill people that they are more than medical patients." Arthur W. Frank, "Enacting Illness Stories: When, What, and Why," in *Stories and Their Limits: Narrative Approaches to Bioethics*, ed. Hilde Lindemann Nelson (New York: Routledge, 1997), 48, n. 15.

8. See Jeffrey P. Bishop, "Creating Narratives in the Clinical Encounter," and Arthur W. Frank, "From Suspicion to Dialogue: Relations of Storytelling in Clinical Encounters," *Medical Humanities Review* 14, no.1 (Spring 2000): 10–23, 24–34.

9. Anne Hunsaker Hawkins, *Reconstructing Illness: Studies in Pathography* (West Lafayette, IN: Purdue University Press, 1993), 161.

10. Ronald A. Carson, "Interpretive Bioethics: The Way of Discernment," *Theoretical Medicine* 11 (1990): 51–59.

11. See, for example, Paul Ricoeur, "The Model of the Text: Meaningful Action Considered as a Text," in *Hermeneutics and the Human Sciences: Essays on Language, Action, and Interpretation*, ed. John B. Thompson (Cambridge: Cambridge University Press, 1981), 197–221, 202–3.

12. Anne Hudson Jones, "Reading Patients—Cautions and Concerns," *Literature and Medicine* 13 (Fall 1994): 194, 195.

13. Anne Hudson Jones, "From Principles to Reflective Practice," in *Philosophy of Medicine and Bioethics: A Twenty-Year Retrospective and Critical Appraisal*, ed. Ronald A. Carson and Chester R. Burns (Dordrecht: Kluwer Academic Publishers, 1997), 194.

14. Walter Benjamin, "The Storyteller," in *Illuminations*, ed. Hannah Arendt and trans. Harry Zohn (New York: Schocken Books, 1985), 83–84.

15. David Hilfiker, "The Case: Clint Wooder," *Second Opinion* 18, no. 2 (October 1992): 43–53.

16. Charles Taylor, "Theories of Meaning," in *Human Agency and Language* (Cambridge: Cambridge University Press, 1985), 248. Subsequent page references to this work appear in parentheses in the text.

17. In an insightful discussion of discourse ethics as a critical philosophical counterpart to narrative ethics, Sally Gadow writes, "Discourse ethics entails relationship between persons who regard each other as moral agents. Their conversation is based on that regard. The relational narrative they compose is an interpretation of their situation together and an imagining of alternatives to which they could both be committed." *Soundings* 78, no. 3/4 (Fall–Winter 1994): 305–6. However, discourse ethics preserves monological agency.

18. "I am trying to call attention here to a common experience. . . . We all know that to say 'thou' to someone presupposes a deep common accord. Something enduring is already present when this word is spoken. When we try to reach agreement on a matter on which we have different opinions, this deeper factor always comes into play, even if we are seldom aware of it." Hans-Georg Gadamer, "The Universality of the Hermeneutical Problem," in *Hermeneutical Inquiry*, vol. 1: *The Interpretation of Texts*, ed. David E. Klemm (Atlanta, GA: Scholars Press, 1986), 182. (Essays originally published in 1966.)

19. Charles Taylor, "The Dialogical Self," in *The Interpretive Turn*, ed. David R. Hiley, James F. Bohman, and Richard Shusterman (Ithaca: Cornell University Press, 1991), 310.

20. Taylor, "Theories of Meaning," 271.

21. Terry Pringle, *This Is the Child* (New York: Alfred A. Knopf, 1983), 69. Subsequent page references to this work appear in parentheses in the text.

22. Martin Buber, "What Is Man?" in *Between Man and Man* (London and Glasgow: The Fontana Library, 1961), 245. (Essay originally published in 1938.)

23. See Arnold van Gennep, *The Rites of Passage* (Chicago: University of Chicago Press, 1960); and Victor W. Turner, "Dewey, Dilthey, and Drama: An Essay in the Anthropology of Experience," in *The Anthropology of Experience*, ed. Victor W. Turner and Edward M. Bruner (Urbana: University of Illinois Press, 1986), 41–42. Also Victor W. Turner, *On the Edge of the Bush: Anthropology of Experience* (Tucson: University of Arizona Press, 1985), 159ff.

24. See Hans-Georg Gadamer, *Truth and Method*, 2nd rev. ed. (New York: Continuum, 1991), 299: "Understanding begins . . . when something addresses us."

CHAPTER 19

NARRATIVE ETHICS, GENE STORIES, AND THE HERMENEUTICS OF CONSENT FORMS
LARRY R. CHURCHILL

O ver the past two decades, the role and status of literary concepts and perspectives in bioethics has flourished and blossomed. In 1980, a few bioethicists were using literature as an interesting way to supplement standard ethical analysis in teaching health science students. But only a fraction of this minority were engaged in a methodological rethinking of the field of bioethics in the light of literature's contributions to understanding the dynamics of human moral experience. Today no one can ignore the importance of literary skills for bioethics or the challenge literary scholars make to philosophy's historical claim to hegemony over ethics more generally. *Narrative ethics* I understand as a term intended in part to capture the contributions that literary methods and perspectives can make—not just to the task of teaching bioethics—but to the tools practitioners bring to the discipline itself.

These contributions have been presented most powerfully and convincingly in three areas: (1) studies devoted to probing the thickness and illuminating the nuance of patients' lives, as represented in their illness narratives; (2) inquiries into medical practice, primarily focused on the relationships between health care professionals and their patients or their patients' families—for example, the way in which patient "histories" and ethics "cases" have been enriched and altered by using literary tools; and, most recently, (3) reflexive looks at bioethics itself in the efforts to interpret its role, status, and meaning as a professional and human enterprise. The essays in this volume are testimony to the vitality of literary ways of thinking and knowing in these three areas.

One of the striking things about this list is its focus on patients and patient care activities. Yet most bioethicists and medical humanities scholars also spend a great deal of their professional lives worrying about human subjects and medical research; for example, serving on institutional review boards (IRBs) and data safety monitoring boards (DSMBs), teaching about research ethics and scientific integrity, or collaborating with clinical investigators. Over the last decade, a substantial percentage of this time has been spent on genetics research. Yet little has been written about how narrative ethics might contribute to our understanding of genetics, medical research in genetics, or human subjects research more generally. My aim in this essay is to begin that conversation.

In making the case that literary modes of interpretation and analysis can have a powerful impact on neglected areas, I put forward two examples, both concerned with genetics. In the first example I will focus on a central image animating genetics research, namely, genetic determinism. I am impressed by the resilience of this image in the thinking of both scientists and the general public despite various disavowals and refutations by scientists themselves and by bioethicists. I will argue that, in correcting the errors of genetic determinism, literary tools may help more than logic does. Considering genetic determinism as a kind of story, with certain appealing features, may help us to break free from it. The second example concerns informed consent or, more precisely, the interpretation of consent forms for gene transfer research. Informed consent has been a perennial preoccupation of bioethicists, so if I can make a case here, it may have broad implications. In both these instances I hope to make evident that the work of ethics is enhanced in a substantial way by literary perspectives.

GENE STORIES

The process of mapping and sequencing the three billion chemical base pairs making up human DNA is nearly complete, and we are now officially in the "postgenomic era."[1] This means that information roughly equivalent to one thousand phone books with one thousand pages each is available for use in confronting the challenge presented by this era: discovering what this vast catalog of information means and how it can be used for human betterment.

Ten years ago, Nobel Prize–winning chemist Walter Gilbert likened the possibilities provided by genomics to a "vision of the Holy Grail" of biology.[2] This is an apt metaphor, considering that the postgenome quest will be a journey marked by moral hazards as well as great promise. Some ethical questions raised in this quest are familiar ones; they concern privacy, confidentiality, and the potential for discrimination in employment, life insurance, and access to health care. Other issues may reverberate more deeply and require tools that are not customarily included in the bioethical repertoire. One of these is less an issue than a way of thinking about genes, a mode of understanding that has profound ethical and social implications. I refer here to genetic determinism.[3]

Genetic determinism is an idea nicely captured by James Watson, who, with Francis Crick, discovered the double helical structure of DNA, and who later became a founding father for the human genome project. According to Watson, we used to believe that our destiny was in the stars, but now we know it is in our genes.[4] The idea that we *are* our genes—that our attitudes, actions, characteristics, and health are fixed in some fundamental and irretrievable way—is the central idea behind genetic determinism.

One of the most persuasive medical examples of this determinism is Huntington's disease. Huntington's is a neurodegenerative disease that typically begins to affect people when they are between the ages of thirty and fifty. If one carries the mutation, disease onset is inevitable in all known environments. There is no prevention, and there is no remedy. Perhaps the best-known person to suffer from Huntington's was Woody Guthrie, whose tragic story was portrayed in the movie *Alice's Restaurant*. The locus of the genetic lesion for Huntington's appears to be the tip of chromosome 4, and the problematic mutation seems to be an abnormally long repetitive chain of the bases cytosine, adenine, and guanine, a so-called CAG repeat. Regardless of other genetic differences or divergent social and physical environments, people with such a mutation are "fixed" on an irreversible course toward debilitation and early death.

The general picture that genetic determinism presents is something like a direct, causal relationship between genotype and phenotype, between a person's genetic constitution and a visible trait, or disease. Huntington's and a few other lesser-known diseases serve as models of the basic idea: genotype *determines* phenotype.

Yet the model for gene function presented in Huntington's is not a typical one. As Philip Kitcher, Jonathan Kaplan, Glenn McGee, and others have pointed out, almost no one in the scientific community openly embraces this simplistic and fatalistic form of genetic determinism.[5] (The forms of genetic determinism entrenched in scientific and public discourse are the more subtle ones as I will illustrate shortly.) Scientists now readily acknowledge that causal links between genes and visible biological traits or diseases are very complex. Indeed, the complexity is staggering. William Gelbart, for example, eschews entirely anything as straightforward as the phone book analogy I cited above. He compares the completion of the human genome project not to reading a phone book or even to finding the Rosetta Stone but to finding the Phaestos Disk—an as yet undeciphered set of glyphs from a Minoan temple.[6] From thinking that each gene produces its own specific protein, we have moved to understanding that each gene can produce multiple proteins, with little or no understanding of what influences the variation or how the proteins interact with each other or with the environment. The mechanisms of biological development are still largely a mystery. Having completed the gene mapping and sequencing task, we are not near the end but near the end of the beginning.

The scientific problem with genetic determinism is its simplicity. Rather than the isomorphic formula—that is, one gene = one trait (or, one gene = one protein = one trait)—the pathways from genes to traits exhibit at least two kinds of heterogeneity. The first is a "clinical heterogeneity."[7] For example, the same genetic mutation in two people can lead to different outcomes. This is true, for example, for phenylketonuria (PKU), a genetic disease that results from the inability to metabolize the amino acid phenylalanine. If untreated, the disease leads to severe retardation. PKU is also an example of a second sort of heterogeneity, "genetic heterogeneity," meaning that different genetic defects can lead to the same clinical outcome. So, although PKU was at one time understood, like Huntington's disease, to be a rather simple embodiment of genetic determinism, the story is currently understood to be more complex.[8] PKU is now largely remediable through a strictly regulated diet. It is hoped that eventually Huntington's, too, will be understood not as an inevitably fatal disease, but as a genetic condition that *if left untreated* leads to a fatal illness.

Yet despite this growing recognition of complexity at one level, simplistic gene stories depicting human essences and origins continue to be part of both the scientific and the popular imagination. Historian of science Evelyn Fox Keller says that the belief that genes contain the determinative, unidirectional force for biological development and that the intra- and intercellular environment—to say nothing of the social environment—can be safely ignored was "the Central Dogma" of biology for the twentieth century.[9] This Dogma, she argues in her most recent book, *The Century of the Gene*, "has become so deeply embedded . . . that it will take far more than good intentions, diligence, or conceptual critique to dislodge it."[10] So even when scientists back away from unidirectional and exclusive causal language and the metaphor of blueprints, they still often talk of genes as "the primary aspects" or "the fundamental units" of life that contain "all the information needed" or "the program" for development. Keller traces this kind of foundational thinking back to the early-twentieth-century work of H. T. Morgan and H. J. Muller, biologists who portrayed the gene as a combination of a "physicist's atom" and a "Platonic soul"—both a building block and an animating force.[11]

In a similar analysis, Kaplan explains that while most scientists are officially antideterministic, much of their work still implicitly assumes that the gene is the natural place to look when attempting to explain, predict, or control traits. Moreover, traits that are thought to be even partially gene related are treated as *primarily* genetic.[12] Thus do genes continue to occupy the central position, and when genetic discoveries are made they are often received by an eager public as confirmation of the Central Dogma that genes have the determinative role in traits and diseases. The list of conditions, diseases, or behaviors identified as possibly caused by genes is very long: a variety of cancers, heart disease, hypertension, alcoholism, hyperactivity, Alzheimer's, stress, risk-taking behaviors, violent tendencies, pyromania, shyness, aggressiveness, homosexuality, and criminality, just to name a few. There are great leaps here, both of logic and imagination, given the relative rarity of single-gene diseases like Huntington's.[13]

Why is the story line of genetic determinism so appealing? One possible reason is the natural human hunger for stories that can encapsulate human origins and essences. The drive for answers to "Why?" questions is powerful, and genetic determinism provides an answer embodied in a powerful and simplistic narrative. Dorothy Nelkin points to the cultural appeal of genetic explanations when she notes that "when E. O. Wilson's *Sociobiology* was published in 1975, *Business Week* ran a series of articles on 'The Genetic Defense of the Free Market.'" Presumably, capitalism is a "natural" state of affairs because it is written into our genes. We are, as it were, "programmed" for it.[14]

Another seductive component of this story is the implication that we may eventually gain control over our destiny. When Watson said our fate is not in the stars but in our genes, he reflected the implicit promise that we will someday cease to be victims and become masters of our destiny. This promise is manifest in the creation of the National Human Genome Research Institute and its heavy investment in gene transfer research, including over four hundred "gene therapy" research protocols over the past decade. It also plays out in the tremendous interest not only in curing disease, but in ambitions to enhance normal human functioning.

Yet there is a darker and more sobering explanation of the appeal of genetic determinism as well. At its worst, the central dogma is an instrument for social repression and political disenfranchisement. It is a dogma not only about how to explain diseases, but how to explain differences in people. The kind of explanations it provides tend to be fatalistic ones, embodying narrative lines that deflect attention from the massive environmental contributions and social forces at work in producing and alleviating diseases and social differences. At its worst, genetic determinism is not only a fatalistic and enervating social philosophy but one that uses biological cover for stigmatization, disenfranchisement, and cultural subjugation. It may appeal to some as a means to merely confirm prejudices about those whom they tend to see as different or defective. In this perverse way, for those who need an ontology to explain their bigotry, the genetic determinism story is comforting.

It is easy to see the hazards of telling the gene story in this way. If genes are the main actors, everything else is reduced to at best a supporting role. For example, if learning difficulties can be explained by genetic deficiencies of the brain, then the vexing and expensive problems of cultural deprivation, nutritional deficits, and impoverished educational environments can be set aside. If lung cancer is best explained by genetic predisposition, then the contentious issues of cigarette advertising, behavioral choices in tobacco use, and the role of environmental and workplace toxins can be put to rest. The assertion that certain races do not perform well in standardized tests because of their educationally inferior genes— essentially the argument of the best-selling book *The Bell Curve*[15]—is yet another hazardous form of genetic determinism that serves to undercut social and political action to remedy inequalities.

Dislodging genetic determinism as the dominant story line is important not only because it is poor science. Of equal or more importance, genetic determinism tends to feed some of our least admirable ambitions for control of our destiny, lodging them in biological causes rather than in social choices; it also plays into some of our most easily perverted fears about difference. In this sense, the story line of genetic determinism could be understood as a replay of the Calvinistic pre-destination narrative, in which the plot is divine preselection for salvation or damnation. Genetic determinism in its crudest form is a kind of biological pre-destination, in which genes take on the role of God's inscrutable pleasure, and medical scientists offering gene therapies play the role of saviors. I don't want to push this analogy too hard. Still, I do want to suggest that it is through recogniz-ing the similarity and sameness among different narratives that we can see why genetic determinism is a story entrenched in our imagination, and also why, in Toni Morrison's words, we don't want to pass this story on.[16]

As I write, a new story about genes seems possible. In the beginning of the human genome project, estimates of the total number of genes in human DNA ran between 80,000 and 100,000. Creatures as complex as we are, it was thought by scientists (working largely from the unidirectional, isomorphic causal para-digm), would require a large number of genes. Now, near the completion of the project, the new estimate of the total number of human genes is between 30,000 and 35,000, only about 50 percent more than a fruitfly or a roundworm and about the same number as corn. Telling this new story about our genes means reassess-ing the foundations of human complexity discussed earlier. But more important, it provides the opportunity for intellectual humility about our understanding of genetic action, for moral caution about loading social and political agendas onto scientific paradigms, and for a new narrative about how to locate ourselves in the natural order.

THE HERMENEUTICS OF CONSENT FORMS

I am a member of a research team at the University of North Carolina that has been at work on informed consent processes for gene transfer research for the past six years.[17] Our most recent area of focus is the concept of benefit. While a great deal of energy has been expended parsing the various meanings of "risk" and try-ing to quantify it accurately, relatively little work has been done on the comple-mentary notion of benefit. Working with categories of benefit such as "direct," "collateral," "societal," and the like, we are in the process of interviewing the sub-jects, investigators, and study coordinators of gene transfer trials, as well as repre-sentatives of the IRBs that oversee them. We are also coding the consent forms for these trials, searching for benefit language in the various sections of these forms, including the purpose, procedures, risks, and alternatives sections as well as the benefits sections. Our overall aim is to develop a composite picture, comparing the understandings of the various players in gene transfer trials. More specific aims are to compare benefit language in a study's protocol with benefit talk in that study's consent form and to assess consent forms for clarity and accuracy in the way benefits are described and discussed. It is in this latter task that important interpretive problems emerge, problems that are best understood and resolved in the idioms of literary criticism.

A few words of background may be helpful at this point. Most gene transfer studies are Phase I trials, namely, studies of safety rather than efficacy. The prospect that a subject in such an early-phase trial will experience personal bene-fit in terms of improved health or greater longevity is usually quite small. For example, in Phase I cancer trials generally, only 4 to 6 percent of subjects experi-ence any benefit, and often this benefit is an improvement measured in scientific terms (for example, tumor shrinkage) rather than an improvement in symptoms or the subject's quality of life.[18] Most clinical trials, even those that reach Phase III, where efficacy is the aim, do not produce major therapeutic breakthroughs. There is as yet no comparable information on the number of subjects who benefit from Phase I gene transfer trials.

Medical researchers remain optimistic about the long-range promise of "gene therapy," but with only ten years of research experience in this field, gene transfer studies are still in their infancy and as yet unsuccessful.[19] Hence, most gene trans-fer consent forms are cautious about promising benefit, especially in the benefit section of these forms. Typically the language is cautious and agnostic: "No bene-fit can be guaranteed from participation in this research," or "We do not know whether you will experience any benefit from this research."

Yet sometimes the language is more direct, stressing the expectations or intentions of researchers: "We do not expect you to benefit personally," or "This research is not designed to cure your disease" (or "improve your condition").

Such language may be accurate or inaccurate, sufficient or insufficient, depending on a wide range of factors. Context is everything. For example, in some trials cautious language that excludes a "guarantee" of benefit could be seen by desperate prospective subjects as implying that a benefit was probable, although not certain. Claims of agnosticism suffer mostly from vagueness and incomplete-ness. They may reflect investigators' honest self-assessments of ignorance about benefits, but they are insufficient and potentially misleading unless modified by statements about probabilities and more specific detail about what sort of bene-fits, if any, might be possible.

Statements about the expectations of investigators and the aims of research usually represent improvements over agnostic disclaimers in the informed con-sent process. Statements that address an investigator's expectations provide sub-jects a window into the investigator's thinking and can enhance the trust elements of a relationship while supplying important information. Statements about the aims of a research project typically signal an improvement of another sort. They allow subjects to better understand, and potentially identify with, the overall research goals—an ethical criterion for research recruitment emphasized by Hans Jonas.[20] Yet identifying with the long-range goals of a line of research must be sep-arated from whatever benefits subjects could realistically expect at the point in the research in which they are involved.

Anyone who has ever served on an IRB knows this set of problems and knows also how IRBs muddle through them, seeking to help investigators provide subjects with as much accurate and clear information as possible. IRBs do not, however, usually think about their task as a hermeneutical enterprise, a task of interpretation raising questions for which literary tools can be helpful.

Consider, for example, the question of *voice* in consent forms.[21] In literary criticism, voice refers to the determinate presence behind all the fictitious voices in a novel, play, or short story. The voice is the authority behind the characters and the story, an agency that selects and renders the literary material in the way in which it appears. In a similar way, investigators embody a voice in their consent forms, creating a story and shaping a plot into which the potential subject is a reader, but a special kind of reader, for the reading constitutes an invitation to literally enter into the story.

But of course investigators are not the only authors, sometimes not even the lead authors, of consent forms. Often the first draft of these stories of research is constructed by pharmaceutical "ghost writers" and presented to investigators along with the protocol. IRBs play their part as well, often inserting prefatory boilerplate language about the general nature of clinical trials or protective language about the limits of institutional liability. Alternatively, the lead author may be an experienced study coordinator with a knack for translating complex science into lay terms. Once written, consent forms are frequently edited and sometimes rewritten by IRB members in their review. Gene transfer protocols are also scrutinized and sometimes reformulated by the Recombinant DNA Advisory Committee. The result can be a refined and more accurate document—or, in the worst cases, an exhibit for Luigi Pirandello's play *Six Characters in Search of an Author*.[22]

The point of asking about voice in any piece of writing is to inquire about the unique human presence behind it. This is, to be sure, no simple task, either in literature or in consent forms. For example, novelists or playwrights may purposefully either deny readers access to a consistent authorial voice or present them with several, seeking to displace or demystify (or mystify) the author's relationship with readers. Yet even in such complex narrative situations, there is the presumption of voice, if only the voice that tries to disabuse readers of a simple and easy access to an author's intentions. In consent forms, asking about voice means seeking the person behind the document, the person authorized to spin a story about the research project and invite subjects to participate in it. Asking about voice moves us beyond the standard questions of risk/benefit ratios and enables us to ask what sort of human contact should be expected from a consent form, and what we can do to help a document elicit and sustain that contact.

It is unfortunate that the interpretation of consent forms as mere vehicles for information is so pervasive; perhaps this is due to the dominance of legal metaphors for consent over moral ones, often resulting in cynicism about the value of consent forms altogether. Attention to elements like voice can help to reawaken awareness that consent forms use language to convey human intentions, goals, and proffered relationships. Language, thus understood, is an instrument for forming, interpreting, and maintaining these relationships, not just a tool for satisfying federal regulators or a formula for legal protection for investigators and institutions. Effacement of the investigator's voice, or imposition of additional voices such that no agency or presence can be discerned, presents an ethical problem even if the consent form conveys accurately the facts and figures about the trial. Attention to voice is a reminder that subjects want and need to know just *who* it is that is speaking to them. Only by identifying the *who* behind the words can subjects begin to discern their own *place* in the research, that is, the meaning of these facts and figures for them as individuals.

Thus, considering voice reveals why casting the discussion of benefits in terms of intentions or research design is usually preferable to general claims of agnosticism or disclaimers about guarantees of benefits. The former say something about the investigator, or the investigator's agency in the project. The latter seem to come from nowhere, speaking from a place disengaged from the ambitions of the research and, more important, disengaged from establishing a relationship with the potential subject.

Let me take this inquiry one step further by asking: In their search for voice and meaning in consent forms, how do subjects read the forms? This became an important issue for our research team as we tried to evaluate gene transfer documents. The aim of any consent form must be to successfully communicate to potential subjects the nature and purpose of the clinical trial, the procedures subjects will undergo, the risks and benefits of participating in the trial, the possible alternatives to enrolling, and so on. Hence, the proper benchmark of interpretation should be what a subject would understand from reading a consent form, not what a scientist might infer from her prior knowledge, and not what an investigator or other author of the forms might be trying to say.

Yet taking subject understanding as the gold standard is no simple matter; neither the forms nor the readers are simple. Consent forms are complex—even on well-defined issues such as benefit—because, as illustrated above, there are many shades of meaning, and for each shade, multiple implications. Moreover, benefit talk is found not only in the section of the consent form designated "Benefits." Benefit language often crops up in descriptions of the "Purpose" of the research, and sometimes in the "Procedures" and also in the "Risks" and "Alternatives" sections. For example, within the "Procedures" section, the insertion of the altered gene product into a subject is often called "the treatment phase" in the research project timeline, and this language can imply to subjects that they are being "treated" for their disease, even when they clearly understand they are enrolled in an early-phase trial. "Purpose" sections are sometimes vehicles for investigators to voice their most ambitious hopes for their research.

The presence of benefit language in various sections of the consent form also raises questions about whether and how to balance the various things that may be said in the form *as a whole* with what is said in the "Benefits" section of the document. For example, it is not unusual to find the prospects for both general, long-term success and for individual subject benefit discussed in specific and optimistic terms in the purpose section, while the "Benefits" section speaks in vague and cautious tones. What do potential subjects make of this? Do they engage in weighing and balancing, sizing up the form as a whole, or do they zero in on certain sections for what they assume to be the authoritative locus for certain issues—for example, looking to the "Benefits" section for the final word on potential benefits? Do subjects read the form as a short story from beginning to end, or do they see these forms as a collection of epigrams, each with its own message? Of course, readers themselves vary in reading style, not to mention level of comprehension, based on expectations, experience in research, background knowledge in science, and a wide variety of other factors.

How can literary concepts and tools help with this task? I will provide only one instance, although I am confident that my literary colleagues could substantially expand the list of examples. In the midst of a long discussion among our research team about how to answer these questions, Nancy King provided, if not the answer, a way to proceed. She said that we are engaged in "reader-response criticism." What she meant, roughly, is that rather than seing the meanings of texts as rather determinate things placed in documents by their authors, we should see the meanings as the production or creation of the individual readers. Although there can be debates about how much of the text is "objectively" given by the author and how much is left to the "subjective" response of a reader, there is always a gap, an irreducible indeterminacy, in texts such that the response element is always present.

This observation is helpful in several ways. First, it helps us to understand the work of IRBs as one of closing the gap of indeterminacy as much as possible, eliminating authors' statements of potential benefits that conflict with the evidence available or are internally inconsistent. If gaps cannot be eliminated entirely, some of the larger or more hazardous ones can at least be spotted and rectified. Second, and more germane to our research, it may be possible to make some reasonable assumptions about the kind of responses subject-readers are likely to make and to assess consent forms based on the extent to which they take these into account. For example, it is evident from several empirical studies that research subjects are vulnerable to "therapeutic misconception," that is, they are likely to overestimate the potential benefit of research participation for themselves.[23] There is, to be sure, a hazard of overgeneralizing the assumptions some reader-subjects may bring to their responses to consent forms. Still, the tendency to read "benefit" into vague or ambiguous statements or to confuse aspirational benefit (long-range promise for future patients) with direct benefit (benefits to the subjects themselves) is well established, so that to fail to note this as a likely reader-response would be a major oversight.

I am not, of course, claiming that IRBs, or even our research team, need to study literary critics associated with "reader-response theory" in order to do their job properly. I am arguing that the availability of such tools and perspectives can make a difference—sometimes a crucial one—in the ways bioethics researchers go about their work. Thinking of potential subjects reading consent forms as reader-responders who are actively constructing meanings as they read is one way that our work can be improved. Taking this seriously as a method for discerning a successful informed consent process might mean that we would spend less time parsing the language of investigators and more time learning about the lived world of subjects in which responses are formed.

And when we do focus on the language that investigators use in consent forms we would do well to give attention to more than reading levels and checklists of required information. Consent forms are narratives in which researchers weave their own hopes for scientific progress and therapeutic advances. A lot has been said about the vulnerability of subjects as readers who often seek more from research participation than can be realistically expected. Attention should also be given to investigators whose vulnerability is sometimes to want more from their research than can be realistically expected. Thinking of consent forms as the written narrative through which investigators and subjects seek to appear and make connection with each other is perhaps our best way of guarding against the confusion between hopes and expectations by both parties.

CONCLUSION

In this essay I have purposively sought to avoid the standard problem list for the utilization of narrative, for example, patients' illness stories and doctor-patient interactions, where the problematic is defined around questions of power and discussed in idioms of autonomy and beneficence. My aim has been to draw attention to areas of ethics work that are usually not discussed as productive fields for narrative approaches, but in which narrative tools and methods can make a real difference. I will have succeeded if other scholars pick up these threads and begin to consider human subjects research and genetics/genomics as areas in which narrative approaches can be fruitfully applied.

NOTES

I thank Nancy King, Gail Henderson, and Michele Easter for their perceptive remarks on earlier drafts of this essay.

1. I owe this phrase to my UNC colleague Terry Magnuson, who also refers to the present era as one of "proteomics," meaning the study of the proteins produced by genes and the changes in protein expression in different environments and conditions.

2. Walter Gilbert, "A Vision of the Grail," in *The Code of Codes*, ed. D. J. Kevles and Leroy Hood (Cambridge, MA: Harvard University Press, 1992), 83–97.

3. I prefer the term *genetic determinism*, but others have discussed this phenomenon as "geneticization." For example, see Ruth Hubbard and Elijah Wald, *Exploding the Gene Myth: How Genetic Information Is Produced and Manipulated by Scientists, Physicians, Employers, Insurance Companies, Educators, and Law Enforcers* (Boston: Beacon Press, 1993), 65–68. A closely related concept is "genetic essentialism," which is expertly described and critiqued by Dorothy Nelkin and M. Susan Lindee in *The DNA Mystique: The Gene as a Cultural Icon* (New York: H. H. Freeman, 1995), 41ff. Nelkin

and Lindee discuss genetic essentialism as a parallel between DNA and the Christian concept of a soul as a personal, individual essence. I think the parallels are actually closer to the classical Greek notion of a soul as found, for example, in Plato, rather than anything distinctive to Christian beliefs, but the idea of DNA as a sacred essence is clear in either case.

4. J. Madeleine Nash and Dick Thompson, "The Gene Hunt," *Time*, March 20, 1999, 62–67.

5. See Philip Kitcher, *The Lives to Come* (New York: Touchstone, 1996); Jonathan Kaplan, *The Limits and Lies of Human Genetic Research* (New York: Routledge, 2000); and Glenn McGee, *The Perfect Baby* (Lanham, MD: Rowman and Littlefield, 1997).

6. Cited in Evelyn Fox Keller, *The Century of the Gene* (Cambridge, MA: Harvard University Press, 2000), 6.

7. Kaplan, *The Limits and Lies of Human Genetic Research*, 18.

8. Ibid., 18ff.

9. Evelyn Fox Keller, *Refiguring Life: Metaphors of Twentieth Century Biology* (New York: Columbia University Press, 1995), 93.

10. Keller, *The Century of the Gene*, 136.

11. Keller, *Refiguring Life*, 9.

12. Kaplan, *The Limits and Lies of Human Genetic Research*, 12ff.

13. In a fascinating editorial, a group from the National Institute for Environmental Health Sciences claims that genetic determinism has led to the "overprotection" of human subjects in research. "The current guidelines reflect an assumption of genetic determinism in which all alleles are expected to have direct and powerful conse-quences on health. In contrast, the common varieties of metabolism genes...are nei-ther necessary nor sufficient to produce disease." Allen J. Wilcox, Jack A. Taylor, Richard R. Sharp, and Stephanie J. London, "Genetic Determinism and the Overprotection of Human Subjects," *Nature Genetics* 21 (1999): 362. While these authors are right about the risk involved in research for self-understanding or familial stigma, there is still a need for confidentiality protections since insurance carriers and companies who review health files, to say nothing of health professionals, may be genetic determinists and practice discrimination. In such cases, it matters little that genetic determinism is bad science and that Wilcox and his colleagues are technically right about overprotection.

14. Dorothy Nelkin, "The Social Power of Genetic Information," in *The Code of Codes*, ed. D. J. Kevles and Leroy Hood (Cambridge, MA: Harvard University Press, 1992), 177–90.

15. Charles Murray and R. J. Herrnstein, *The Bell Curve* (New York: The Free Press, 1994).

16. Toni Morrison, *Beloved* (New York: Alfred A. Knopf, 1987), 275.

17. This work includes two separate but related projects funded by the National Human Genome Research Institute, through its Ethical, Legal, and Social Issues Program. Both projects concern issues of informed consent in gene transfer research. I was PI for the first project, and my colleagues Gail Henderson and Nancy King are co-PIs for the second, which runs through 2003.

18. See Christopher Daugherty et al., "Perceptions of Cancer Patients and Their Physicians Involved in Phase I Trials," *Journal of Clinical Oncology* 13 (1995): 1062–72.

19. Even calling such trials "gene therapy" research can be misleading, both to subjects and to investigators. See Larry R. Churchill, Myra L. Collins, Nancy M. P. King, Stephen G. Pemberton, and Keith A. Wailoo, "Genetic Research as Therapy:

Implications of 'Gene Therapy' for Informed Consent," *Journal of Law, Medicine and Ethics* 26 (1998): 38–47.

20. Hans Jonas, "Philosophical Reflections on Experimenting with Human Subjects," *Daedalus* 98, no. 2 (Spring 1969): 235ff.

21. For a concise summary of the notion of voice in literature see M. H. Abrams, *A Glossary of Literary Terms* (New York: Holt, Rinehart, and Winston, 1999), 218ff. Attention to "voice" in consent forms leads naturally to an exploration of "voices," meaning looking of multiple persona, intentions, and agendas, as well as to "different voices," in the sense of Carol Gilligan's landmark volume, *In a Different Voice: Psychological Theory and Women's Development* (Cambridge, MA: Harvard University Press, 1982). Those acquainted with human subjects research recognize that the reasons subjects give for enrolling in clinical trials often revolve around relationships— for example, loyalties to one's fellow sufferers in a cancer support group, or responsibilities to one's children—when a genetic component is involved. More generally, understanding research participation as relationally motivated would help to show the deficiencies in looking at consent forms simply as documents that disclose information, and why locating the voice, or voices, is important.

22. Luigi Pirandello, "Six Characters in Search of an Author," in *Naked Masks*, ed. Eric Bentley (New York: E. P. Dutton, 1952).

23. P. S. Appelbaum, L. R. Roth, and C. Lidz, "The Therapeutic Misconception: Informed Consent in Psychiatric Research," *International Journal of Law and Psychiatry* 5 (1982): 319–29. See also Churchill, et al., "Gene Research as Therapy."

CHAPTER 20

NARRATIVE, ETHICS, AND PAIN:
THINKING *WITH* STORIES
DAVID B. MORRIS

No moral theory can be adequate if it does not take into account the narrative character of our experience.

— *Mark Johnson,* Moral Imagination

I s it possible that ethical action might depend less on analytical reasoning than on responding to a dilemma as we might respond to a story? "Thinking with stories" is a concept I borrow from sociologist Arthur W. Frank in *The Wounded Storyteller.*[1] By "thinking," Frank means and I mean a process very different from the exclusive operation of reason. Thought clearly involves reasoning, in addition to various forms of cognitive activity from memory to meditation, but I want to emphasize that thinking also involves a crucial collaboration with feeling. In fact, the ancient Western binary habit that requires us to put reason and emotion into separate words and unconnected categories is, I contend, a neurological mistake, with crucial implications for ethics. We need a greatly revised understanding of reason and emotion—a revision consistent with recent discoveries in cognitive science—in order to escape the history of erroneous assumptions about thinking and about ethics, a history that I wish to challenge. The concept of thinking with stories is meant to oppose and modify (not replace) the institutionalized Western practice of thinking about stories. Thinking about stories conceives of narrative as an object. Thinker and object of thought are at least theoretically distinct. Thinking with stories is a process in which we as thinkers do not so much work on narrative as take the radical step back, almost a return to childhood experience, of allowing narrative to work on us.

I. INTRODUCTION: THE CALL OF NARRATIVE

Let me be clear. It makes no sense to challenge an erroneous split between reason and emotion by installing an ironclad, artificial division between thinking about stories and thinking with stories. Thinking with stories likely constitutes for some people a stage—possibly an indivisible stage—in a dynamic, dialectical, dialogical process that includes thinking about stories. The process of thinking with stories, however, is so thoroughly neglected, even within the field of reader-response theory, that my aim is to explore its power to take us beyond the usual academic traditions of narrative analysis and to put us in contact with valuable resources for moral thought and action. Anthropologist Keith H. Basso in *Wisdom Sits in Places* shows how Apache people in the U.S. Southwest live today in a local world richly endowed with narrative meaning—where the reference to specific places (such as Line-of-White-Rocks or Red-Ridge-with-Alder-Trees) instantly evokes tales of what happened there. In a culture that avoids direct rebuke, these narratives, as Basso demonstrates, provide unobstrusive and gentle but steady moral guidance. One Apache male describes how such tales, when retold in the context of moral misconduct, have a way of almost literally getting under your skin: "That story is working on you now. You keep thinking about it. That story is changing you now, making you want to live right. That story is making you want to replace yourself."[2]

The stunning concept of stories that make you want to replace yourself might be said to underwrite an entire ethics of narrative. Stories from this perspective are not detached fictions or casual entertainment but, as among the Cashinahua Indians of the upper Amazon, experiences that incur an obligation on the listener.[3] Such stories exert a kind of "call." The moral call of stories is hardly restricted to indigenous traditions or to peoples in remote locations. Harvard psychiatrist Robert Coles has described how stories exercise a moral force in the lives of his patients and students in contemporary Cambridge.[4] A small band of philosophers from Aristotle to Iris Murdoch has staked a claim for stories in engaging what we might call the moral imagination, and there is even an emerging scholarly literature devoted to "narrative ethics."[5] Ample precedent thus exists for challenging the dominant approach that regards narrative as either value-free products of the entertainment industry or as complex objects of analytical interpretation (sometimes both at once). My question is how such a challenge might engage the neglected, often moral, and always more than strictly rational processes by which stories work on us.

Until recently, readers conventionally understood stories as divided into separate and nonoverlapping types: fiction and nonfiction. Nonfictional stories purported to stake truth claims about characters and events, while fiction (even if imitating nonfiction) belonged in a realm of the made-up, imagined, or patently untrue. Contemporary blends of fact and invention—from new journalism to virtual reality—have thoroughly eroded such conventional distinctions. The articles in *JAMA* differ in obvious ways from a pulp novel, but differences clear at the extremes help call attention to the vast unclear intermediate range where nonfiction mingles with fiction and where life is increasingly drawn into the artful orbit of story. "News magazines present the events of the world as an ongoing weekly serial," novelist E. L. Doctorow observes. "Weather reports are constructed on television with exact attention to conflict (high pressure areas clashing with lows), suspense (the climax of tomorrow's weather prediction coming after the commercial), and other basic elements of narrative." Reflecting on the relentless appropriation of fictional techniques by people who create, advertise, package, and market "factual products," Doctorow concludes, "I am thus led to the proposition that there is no fiction or nonfiction as we commonly understand the distinction: there is only narrative."[6] Narrative in its power to swallow up distinctions between fiction and nonfiction reminds us how far medicine now constitutes a nonstop cascade of dramatic events and gripping revelations, from soap operas to congressional hearings. An absorbing medley of scientific studies are reported on TV newscasts—transformed into what journalists call "stories"—days before they appear in medical journals. Today medicine and human health fall inexorably, sooner or later, under the spell of narrative.

Pain is nearly as immeasurable as narrative, and in examining the possibilities of a narrative ethics I will focus on pain specifically within medicine.[7] This focus seems appropriate because pain in the developed world has been thoroughly medicalized, and medicine has worked out a very specific relation to pain. There is even a new specialty known as pain medicine, in which doctors rely upon a bedrock clinical and theoretical distinction between two very different kinds of pain: acute and chronic.[8] (Acute and chronic pain differ significantly enough that they require very different therapies.) In addition, medicine has achieved the near miracle of consensus on a working definition. The International Association for the Study of Pain (IASP)—the authoritative scientific and medical organization—defines pain as "an unpleasant sensory and emotional experience associated with actual or potential tissue damage, or described in terms of such damage."[9] A quiet revolution is at work within this somewhat bland account. The IASP invokes the traditional one-to-one link between pain and tissue damage only to reconfigure the connection as a loose network of possibilities. Tissue damage alone is no longer a prerequisite for pain. In one study, half the subjects reported pain when attached to a stimulator set to produce, without their knowledge, nothing beyond a low humming sound.[10] Moreover, the IASP definition describes pain not only as a sensory phenomenon but also, in an historic shift, as an emotional experience. Emotion is now regarded as intrinsic to pain, not merely a response or separable add-on. Pain specialist Mark D. Sullivan, recuperating the view of Aristotle, goes so far as to title an article "Pain as Emotion."[11] Finally, in an objectivity-busting footnote to their definition, the IASP insists that pain is "always subjective" and "always a psychological state."[12] The object of study, if you are studying pain, is no longer an object. Ethicists and narratologists need not uncritically adopt this new understanding of pain, but they would be unwise to ignore it.

Ethics, like pain, has also found a special niche within medicine in recent years, and a new professional discipline called bioethics began to emerge in the 1970s. The dominant approach in bioethics quickly became known as principlism—an offspring of the Enlightenment tradition in which human reason discovers, formulates, and applies a system of universally binding moral standards.[13] Principlism in bioethics is inseparable from its four big guns—autonomy, beneficence, nonmaleficence, and justice—often invoked as moral absolutes that contain the solution to any medical dilemma. This four-principle approach has found wide acceptance within medicine, and it is hard to imagine how ethics can survive a complete absence of principle. The question is how principles are regarded. The convincing arguments against principlism do not reject principles but reject the claim that principles hold absolutist status as expressions of universal reason. Properly understood, as Mark Johnson writes from a perspective of cognitive semantics, principles are "crystallizations of the insights that emerge out of a people's ongoing experience."[14] A bioethics today that focused solely on stories—oblivious to the crystallizations of principle—would not only run afoul of the hard-won medical consensus in favor of the four-principle approach. It would also fail to offer the protections necessary in a profession where money and power always place the patient at risk. If bioethics needs principles, however, it is also starting to find unprecedented uses for narrative, and narrative within bioethics is starting to shed its former status as little more than a synonym for anecdote or falsehood.[15] What follows are three exploratory probes (to use a space-age term) into the changing relations among ethics, narrative, and pain. The probes are not meant to build up an argument but, in exploratory fashion, to advance an understanding—inside and outside medicine—of what it might mean to think *with* stories.

II. A BIOCULTURAL MODEL

The three exploratory probes will make most sense set within a framing distinction between what in *Illness and Culture in the Postmodern Age* I call modern and postmodern illness.[16] Illness in the modern era was keyed to the grand narrative of the biomedical model. As George L. Engel argued in a famous essay published in *Science,* the biomedical model during the early twentieth century rapidly achieved the status of dogma, constituting not only the dominant scientific model of disease but also the dominant folk model.[17] Almost everybody bought into it. Engel describes the biomedical model as dualistic, mechanistic, and reductive: that is, it divides bodies from minds, it understands bodies on analogy with machines, and it reduces biological processes to a language of chemistry and physics. This model of modern illness needs revision when applied to specific disciplines—family practice and surgery do not share identical views—but it will strike many patients as remarkably accurate. Postmodern illness, by contrast, although it never rejects the discoveries of science or wholly breaks free from the power of the biomedical model, encompasses a recognition that disease and illness are often inseparably linked with culture. From stress, sedentary lifestyles, and poor diet to environmental toxins, the forces that underlie many forms of organic dysfunction are social and psychological. Illness, we are now coming to recognize, is not solely the result of bodily mechanisms gone awry but an experience constructed at the crossroads of biology and culture.

The construction of illness at the crossroads of biology and culture illustrates the process of "double-coding" that architectural historian Charles Jencks described as a distinctive trait of postmodernism. Jencks defines double-coding in postmodern architecture as "the combination of Modern techniques with something else (usually traditional building)."[18] The former AT&T Building—now the Sony Building—in New York City has subsequently attained almost celebrity status as an instance of postmodern double-coding: a typical modernist glass box that culminates in a Chippendale roofline. In medicine, however, a very similar process of double-coding applies as American patients continue to consult their Western doctors while simultaneously paying huge out-of-pocket sums for non-traditional therapies.[19] It also underlies increasingly hybrid approaches, as reflected in *The Scalpel and the Silver Bear*, where, as the dust jacket puts it, "the first Navajo woman surgeon combines Western medicine and traditional healing."[20] The magnitude of change is also reflected in a graph based on figures that show the growth of per-capita expenditure for health care in America during the period generally called postmodern (figure 20.1).[21]

The steep upward slope attests to the postmodern alteration of illness from a biomedical to a biocultural condition: it acknowledges the emergence of powerful cultural forces from mass media and government subsidies to multinational drug companies. A biocultural model recognizes how inextricably we are situated inside the new network of medical consumerism. Health (or an appearance of health) has become a prized commodity, as proudly displayed as a new SUV, while illness is an evil warded off with multivitamins and gym memberships. One additional index of change is the political and social conflict that follows a focus on the cultural construction of illness, as, for example, when public health organizations vigorously promote safe sex while AIDS activists attack the Roman Catholic Church over its position against homosexuality. The revelation of how far the biology of affliction is influenced by cultural events also contains a promise that we may come to understand how illness can be crucially modified or wholly reconstructed by its contact with narrative.

Pain, too, is changed within this biocultural postmodern landscape. Neurosurgeon John Loeser, former president of the American Pain Society, describes pain (specifically chronic pain) as distinct from the mechanical activity of nerves and neurotransmitters that specialists call nociception. Loeser's account drastically revises the biomedical, nerve-centered account of pain. "The brain," he writes, "is the organ responsible for all pain." This statement suggests a profound redirection of research and treatment. "All sensory phenomena, including nociception," Loeser adds, "can be altered by conscious and unconscious mental activity."[22] The hottest area of research today focuses on the brain and on cortical representations of pain.[23] The brain that Loeser invokes, moreover, is no Cartesian screen passively receiving data from the senses but a conscious, active, Janus-like power looking both inward and outward: inward as it monitors and adjusts bodily processes but also, crucially, outward, as it connects us with the interpersonal world of human culture. We know that ethnicity influences pain.[24] Gender influences pain.[25] So do other complicated mixes of national, religious, and cultural background. Chronic low back pain patients in Japan, for example, proved to be

FIGURE 20.1 Aggregate Private and Public Health Expenditures in the U.S.

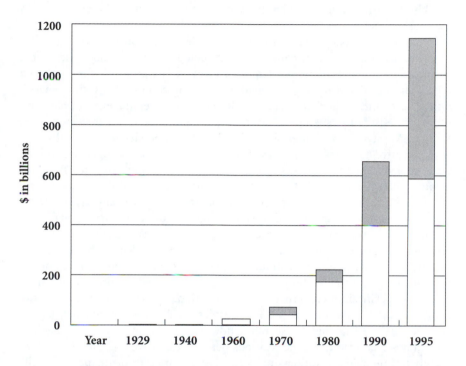

Data Source: Knickman and Thorpe, "Financing for Healthcare," in *Jonas's Health Care Delivery in the United States*, ed. Anthony R. Kovner et al., 5th ed. (New York: Springer, 1995), 268. Graphics courtesy of Frances Kelleher. Darker bar = public health expenditure. Lighter bar = private health expenditure.

significantly less impaired—in psychological, social, vocational, and avocational function—than similar patients in America.[26] In short, postmodern pain is no longer officially divided along Cartesian lines that put it into separate boxes labeled physical and mental. It is, even if not usually described this way, a biocultural event, subject to both individual and transpersonal modulation, as variable across social boundaries as other events with mixed biological and cultural significance, from childbearing to suffering.[27] Pain, in short, has been remade as irreversibly open to the hubbub of human social and psychic life and thus open to an inescapable intersection with narrative.

Narrative, like pain, takes on new features in the era of postmodern illness when culture enters into new commerce with biology. Under the old regime of the biomedical model, narrative was largely irrelevant. The patient's story, as Frank argued in *The Wounded Storyteller*, had no standing compared with the doctor's official, scientific, authoritative account. Recently, however, the place of narrative in medicine is being redefined from multiple perspectives.[28] In *Doctors' Stories*, Kathryn Montgomery Hunter shows how medical knowledge is shot through with narrative, from traditional case histories to anecdotes swapped around the water cooler.[29] The growing persuasiveness of this view is suggested in a 1998 collection (published by the British Medical Journal Press) entitled *Narrative Based Medicine*.[30] The title openly invites comparison with the statistically based practice now entrenched in hospitals and research programs under the name "evidence-based" medicine. Empirical evidence also suggests, however, that narrative holds remarkable therapeutic promise. James W. Pennebaker and Sandra K. Beall found that writing in narrative form about trauma was associated with various health benefits, while Joshua M. Smyth and colleagues showed significant symptom reduction specifically among rheumatoid arthritis patients who wrote in narrative form about stressful experiences.[31] Such studies usually warn about small sample size and the need for more research. Under the old regime of the biomedical model, however, studies on the relations between narrative and illness were not merely unfundable but unimaginable. Today narrative in medicine, especially among researchers who employ ethnographic methods, has not fully unpacked its bags, but it has definitely arrived.

Pain in the postmodern era has entered into a new relation with narrative, which includes a new awareness of its earlier narrative representations.[32] Each best-seller list includes books by people struggling with afflictions from arthritis to zoster. Not only has pain created a fresh alliance with traditional forms of narrative, but narrative discourse about pain has spilled over into such novel public spaces as support groups and Internet chat rooms. The change goes beyond giving the patient's story a respectful hearing. Pain is now understood as "interpersonal."[33] It can no longer be contained wholly within the individual nervous system. Research into "pain beliefs"—specific cognitive-emotional attitudes expressed or embodied by patients—offers a well-documented instance of how knowledge and values within a culture shape the individual experience of pain.[34]

In a study of one hundred patients, such beliefs and attitudes about pain correlated directly with treatment outcomes.[35] A small industry now explores the slippery ways in which pain finds psychosocial sources and complications in cultural systems near and far, from families to disability insurance.[36] Your likelihood of suffering chronic back pain is directly related to your job satisfaction.[37] The response of other people can modify the pain from a condition even so obviously organic as spinal cord injury.[38] This biocultural frame does not deny that biological processes underlie pain. Biology and culture, however, interact in complex, unstable ratios. What matters is to recognize that we are living through a major shift in thinking about pain and that the change from a biomedical to a biocultural model, with its confusing double-coded combinations, holds serious consequences for the changing relations among pain, ethics, and narrative.

III. PAIN AND ETHICS: TWO PROBES

Recently I attended a medical school symposium on pain and ethics. I won't tell the whole story, but the varied if somewhat predictable procession of medical speakers concluded with the chair of anesthesiology. He spoke gravely and precisely about the burdensome demands on his budget and staff, citing multiple troubles that included university cutbacks in funding and state directives about mandatory care for the poor. His solemn and measured tones left me unprepared for his sweeping conclusion. When it comes to the treatment of pain in his department, he stated, "It is no longer possible to do the right thing."

The statement offers a revealing glimpse into the ethics of postmodern medicine. The speaker is postmodern not in expressing doubt, irony, relativism, or indeterminacy. He assumes that he knows what the right thing is, and he knows, with equal conviction, that it is simply impossible to do. The impasse seems distinctively postmodern because it resists a solution through principles or reason alone. The impersonal construction ("it is no longer possible") suggests that this particular medical quandary is not about the failure of specific moral agents but about the insignificance of individual moral agency. The problem is less with persons than with their relation to an amorphous, impersonal, unfixable system. An ethics responsive to such distinctively postmodern dilemmas may need tools as unthinkable within traditional biomedicine as studies on the relations between narrative and arthritis pain. In his confession of powerlessness, the speaker identifies a point where medicine needs to take seriously the understanding that ethics involves more than principles: it also involves, as ethicists are beginning to recognize, stories.[39]

Philosopher Alasdair McIntyre, writing on moral theory, articulates a now widely shared belief when he describes humankind as "essentially a story-telling animal." He adds: "we all live out narratives in our lives" and "we understand our own lives in terms of the narratives that we live out."[40] These narratives of personal identity often reproduce (or crash into) concealed social narratives, with major ethical consequences. Like most developed nations, for example, Scandinavian countries face rapidly mounting claims for pain associated with automobile accidents. Lithuania, however, which has no auto insurance, also shows no significant difference between accident victims and a control group in reports of headache and neck pain.[41] Chronic whiplash syndrome is at least partly an artifact of social narratives about automobile insurance. It is the narrative, as much as the accident or neuron, that produces the neck pain. A similar thought lies behind the 1995 report, from a prestigious IASP task force, entitled *Back Pain in the Workplace*. Chronic back pain in the absence of an organic lesion, it contends, should no longer be classified a medical problem eligible for disability status but reclassified as "activity intolerance." [42] Activity intolerance in effect is less a diagnosis than a counter-narrative meant to contest the cultural script that allows certain patients to redeem their chronic pain for government cash and for freedom from job obligations. (It is a script that entails large social costs and that makes successful medical treatment more difficult.[43]) The pain narratives that we live out today—narratives not entirely of our own making—exist inside a distinctive postmodern landscape that establishes careers for patients potentially as confining and damaging as the ethically obtuse, male-directed narrative of hysteria in the nineteenth century.

A narrative ethics, in exposing intended and unintentional damage to patients, must be willing to pose hard questions. Are authorities right to withhold financial aid simply because a specific historical narrative of disability insurance appears to make medical treatment more difficult? Is activity intolerance merely a euphemism within a concealed social narrative that seeks to lower the cost of public assistance by rejecting patients for whom a doctor cannot find lesions corresponding to their pain? Medicine, however, can pose equally awkward questions. What is the value of narrative practices always open to a conflict of interpretations or to a potentially undecidable proliferation of meanings? Unlike literary theorists, doctors are vulnerable every day to litigation for malpractice, and the last thing they need in facing difficult ethical decisions is an unstoppable freeplay of indeterminacies. Medicine is a practical discipline that values useful information. The value of narrative bioethics may lie precisely in its power to illuminate the submerged struggles native to every local world where moral action, for doctors as for patients, is lived out under the spell of story.

Probe two concerns a story reported in the *New York Times* about a California Medicaid patient, Mrs. Ozzie Chavez.[44] Mrs. Chavez was refused a fairly standard form of anesthesia in labor because she hadn't paid an additional and illegal fee demanded in advance by the anesthesiologist. Such demands, the article says, were somewhat common in light of California's substandard Medicaid reimbursement policies, so this is not just another "horror story" (to cite an unofficial medical genre popular on talk and news shows) about renegade doctors. Mrs. Chavez's experience offers more than a troubling snapshot of pain treatment in postmodern America. It also exposes the often piously concealed American social narrative in which health care is equivalent to cash. "The anesthesiologist wouldn't even come into the room until she got her money," the *Times* reports Mrs. Chavez as saying. "I was lying there having contractions, and they wouldn't give me an epidural. I felt like an animal."

Narrative bioethics will not get us to the bottom of this event—to expose the truth about what really happened in Mrs. Chavez's room—but it helps unfold the implications of her experience. For example, a recognition of the constructedness of all narrative—including the *Times* report—reminds us that Mrs. Chavez's story might have unfolded differently in countries with universal health care, with different patterns of analgesia use, or with different cultural attitudes toward pain in childbirth. Narrative bioethics also directs us to consider the novelistic clash of voices, dialects, and values. The American Society of Anesthesiologists ran an account about Mrs. Chavez in its newsletter that elicited the following response from one of its members: "Poor people can't expect to drive a Rolls Royce, so why should they expect to receive the Cadillac of analgesics for free?" As if to head off a looming public relations disaster, the president of the American Society of Anesthesiologists, John B. Neeld, Jr., shifted deftly from medical car-talk to a language of principles. "It is unethical," he asserted, invoking the principle of beneficence with the certainty of a player snapping down the ace of trumps, "to withhold services because of reimbursement."[45] End of story?

A narrative bioethics—as distinguished from analysis seeking to establish facts—would not consider the case closed when one character implicitly denounces the view of another character as unethical. Characters in fiction denounce each other, explicitly, all the time. Because all stories include gaps, narrative bioethics would stress how little we know about Neeld, Mrs. Chavez, and the unnamed female anesthesiologist. It would remind us to examine not only what is said but also what remains unsaid or even unsayable.[46] Neeld doesn't say—is it unsayable?—that medical services are withheld every day in America because of inability to pay. Sixteen percent of the U.S. population has no health insurance.[47] Services for pain are also routinely withheld for reasons apparently unconnected with ability to pay. A prominent study showed that 50 percent of dying hospitalized patients spent at least half their time, according to family members, in moderate to severe pain.[48] A follow-up study conducted after the hospitals spent six months trying to improve this dismal record showed no change whatever. Information about medical undertreatment for pain has been available to doctors for over twenty-five years, and it has made no impact on improving pain treatment.[49] Clearly, the ethical implications of medical undertreatment for pain remain widely ignored or invisible—at least until narrative, as in the case of Mrs. Chavez, suddenly thrusts pain and its discontents into the headlines.

The persistent, widespread medical undertreatment of pain provides a telling instance of the narratives submerged throughout the experience of postmodern illness. It exposes an unacceptable story in which the pain of certain people—for example, the "dramatically undertreated" pain of AIDS patients—is held of no account.[50] Medicine defaults toward inadequate pain treatment partly because doctors fear state and national drug enforcement agencies, much as they worry over licensing and disciplinary boards.[51] Medical schools also generally fail to offer a pain curriculum.[52] Anxiety is thus compounded by unacknowledged ignorance that strives to preserve the most treasured of modernist icons: the wise physician. Nor can doctors escape their surrounding culture with its contradictory narratives about pain, drugs, gender, and race. Race, for example, has a seldom-discussed relation to the pain of sickle-cell disease, as sickle-cell disease in the United States affects mainly African Americans. Their emergency-room requests for pain medication have a silent history of dismissal by hospital staff (heeding nonmedical social narratives) as drug-seeking behavior.[53] Race even bars access to pain relief by patients who hold valid prescriptions. In New York City, pharmacies in white neighborhoods are three times more likely than pharmacies in nonwhite neighborhoods to carry adequate supplies of opioid analgesics.[54] Mrs. Chavez's troubles have everything to do with her socioeconomic status, if not with her Hispanic surname. Language, including the barriers that it creates for non-native speakers, is as important to narrative bioethics as the social landscape that it reflects. We should notice that Mrs. Chavez didn't say she felt pain. She said she felt like an animal. Unlike Neeld's invocation of principle, her blunt words address a hands-on everyday ethics of respect and degradation. It brings moral theory down to earth, where nonwhites can't get adequate pain medication at their local drugstores while well-paid administrators hold forth on beneficence.

Narrative does not necessarily tell us who is right or wrong. In fact, it actively undermines the false confidence—born of absolutist, objectivist theories of morality—that an ethical dilemma necessarily calls for or accommodates a single right action. What narrative offers to bioethics are means to enhance understanding of the multiple values and conflicting perspectives at stake in medical action or inaction. It offers to situate moral thought within a form of understanding that finds stories as valuable, in their own way, as statistics. Narrative is as relevant to bioethics, for example, as the wildly uneven figures for worldwide prescription of morphine, in which mere statistics cannot tell us about the innumerable patients in Mexico whose double-coded pain has less to do with biology or neuroscience than with the U.S. war against drug traffickers.[55] When we possess financial and technical means of relief, failure to relieve pain comes dangerously close to deliberately inflicting it. Doctors and politicians, however, are not alone in ignoring an ethics of pain. Bioethics has long avoided the problem of medical undertreatment.[56] Principles, it appears, are not enough. A bioethics that addresses the international failure to provide adequate relief for pain requires something like the resources of narrative to reveal both the suffering that statistics always conceal and the complexly interwoven texture of responsibility that makes adequate relief of pain so difficult to obtain. It would need to confront the recognition that pain is not just a medical or neurological problem but implacably biocultural.

IV. THE GREAT MOMENT

The two preceding probes explore the ways in which pain often places patients and caregivers in positions of ethical dilemma. A final probe challenges the still prevalent (modernist) account of pain as a private, interior state—knowable only to the person who feels it, even then bereft of language, and ultimately incommunicable. To the contrary, although pain is always subjective and never fully communicable, it also belongs to social and interpersonal codes as intelligible as "SOS." We may not be able to answer every SOS, but it is self-deception to pretend that we have no idea what it means or what response it asks. Pain, like narrative, exerts an implicit call or obligation. Stories, in addition, can reveal much about the social meanings, public beliefs, and shared codes often inseparable from the individual's experience of pain.[57] For centuries people understood their pain within narrative contexts that explained affliction as divine punishment, even as many people today automatically understand their pain within a reductive and outmoded modernist biomedical narrative concerned solely with damaged tissue or misfiring neurons. What usually goes unnoticed—what I would like to emphasize here—is the relationship that connects pain with narrative meanings and with the emotion they frequently entail.

Narratives work on us, with some clear exceptions, partly by engaging emotion—one reason why Plato banished artists from his ideal republic—and an epoch-making revaluation of emotion is currently under way in disciplines from education and women's studies to psychoanalysis.[58] This revaluation reaches into medicine through a new concern for empathy. [59] Mostly, however, emotion remains a neglected resource in bioethical thought. It may be neglected partly because emotion is double-edged and dangerous. Nazi Germany showed how nationalist narratives of racial purity can mobilize feeling for vicious ends, much as the biblical story of the Good Samaritan enlists emotion on the side of virtue. Still, while emotion is no guarantee of right action, neither is it synonymous with irrationality and error. We must emphatically reject the ancient myth that emotion is a primitive wild-man or wild-woman within, fundamentally antithetical to thought. From road rage to spouse abuse, emotion flows through channels of cultural thinking that underwrite or permit certain kinds of behavior. A man beats his wife not only because he feels angry but also because he believes he can get away with it. We help an enemy not only because we feel compassion but also because we know the story of the Good Samaritan. It will not work to picture emotion as the feral horse running away with reason. The emotion implicit in narrative provides a valuable resource, I contend, in the formation of moral knowledge and of ethical action.

The ethical relations among narrative, emotion, and pain intersect in a fascinating film by the distinguished Hollywood writer and director Preston Sturges. *The Great Moment* (1944) is a little-known biopic that centers on William Morton and his role in the mid-nineteenth-century invention of surgical anesthesia.[60]

Morton supplied both the ether and the expertise that chief surgeon John Collins Warren relied upon in the first public demonstration of pain-free surgery. October 14, 1846, at Massachusetts General Hospital was a day when the world truly changed forever. Ether both delivered patients from the monstrous pain of surgery without anesthesia and permitted doctors to develop slower, more intricate operations impossible with fully conscious patients. As with other breakthroughs, controversy soon embroiled Morton's claims to scientific honor. The film in fact begins with a flashforward that shows Morton worn out with poverty, frustration, and continual setbacks in his efforts to achieve recognition. The ethical impact of the film depends partly on knowing that Morton died a ruined man.

Probe three concerns the conclusion to *The Great Moment*. While crowds throng outside Mass General in anticipation of the world's second pain-free operation, behind closed doors a delegation from the Massachusetts Medical Society meets with Warren, the patriarchal chief surgeon who will again perform the operation. They have arrived to lodge an official protest against further operations, on the ethical ground that physicians are forbidden to employ medicines whose ingredients are unknown: a rule designed to protect patients from quacks and based on the Hippocratic principle of do no harm (or nonmaleficence). The protest occurs because Morton has disguised his discovery under the classical name Letheon in order to keep its ingredients secret. His dilemma is that you can't patent ether. As a means to secure his financial interests, he has applied to patent an ether inhaler—crucial in administering the proper dose—but the patent is still ungranted. What complicates this encounter is the obvious disdain that the upper-class physicians of the Massachusetts Medical Society feel for Morton, a lowly dentist. Thus, while the principle they invoke is clear, its application in Morton's case is deeply compromised. Morton faces an irreconcilable choice. Fortune and fame seem assured if he refuses a premature disclosure of Letheon. A refusal, however, means that an unknown patient must undergo a harrowing leg amputation performed, as Warren puts it matter-of-factly, "in the old way." Morton hesitates. Warren yields to the protest of his colleagues, rejecting the offer of Letheon, and proceeds to the nearby surgical theater.

The camera, in a lingering portrait of his isolation and indecision, follows Morton as he walks slowly down a long empty hallway, holding the useless ether inhaler like a wounded bird. The Ave Maria plays softly in the background as a priest ministers to the young patient lying on a stretcher outside the closed doors of the operating theater. As the priest departs, Morton ends his long walk at the stretcher. He mumbles a few words of concern to the girl who awaits the amputation of her leg. No one has told her that the use of Letheon has been blocked. In response to Morton's concern, she tells him (one big tear glistening on her cheek) that a gentleman has made a new discovery and that the operation doesn't hurt anymore. Morton pauses. The irony of her false confidence and of his complicity in her unanticipated, imminent pain hangs bitterly in the air. Then, in a burst of emotion, he decides. The secret of Letheon will be revealed. The girl will have immediate access to surgical anesthesia. As if in concert with his decision, the doors of the operating theater fling open, light floods the space, and a stirring crescendo swells to its climax as "The End" (meaning here, all's right with the world) flashes on the screen.

The film leaves no doubt about what constitutes Morton's great moment. It is not the world-changing scientific demonstration of surgical anesthesia. In the narrative that Sturges creates, Morton's truly great moment is the instant of ethical decision when he risks his legitimate self-interest and the future of his family so that one anonymous patient will be spared immense unnecessary pain. We already know that this decision will ruin him. More important, we have learned that the choice to relieve or not to relieve pain always has ethical implications: knowledge lost, as we have seen, to many doctors today. Edmund Pellegrino, a giant of contemporary bioethics, asserted recently that not to relieve pain optimally is "tantamount to moral and legal malpractice."[61] *The Great Moment* grounds this insight not in principle or in the threat of legal action but in a direct encounter between doctor and patient, with its inescapable possibility of emotion. The emotion and its ethical implications are what I want to explore in asking how Sturges's narrative works on us.

The ethical implications of emotion for bioethics are crucial especially because medicine engages in a legendary devaluation of feeling (justified often in the name of objectivity). Physician and writer Rafael Campo describes his own medical training as a period when concern for one's emotional life—as opposed to memorizing facts—constitutes almost a breach of professional ethics.[62] Most textbooks in bioethics are nothing if not a dense web of reasoning. Indeed, emotion is so undervalued (if not feared and reviled) in most medical contexts that it is useful to consider philosopher Martha Nussbaum when she argues that emotion is vital to the creation of ethical knowledge. She draws her argument, pertinently, from Greek narrative. "Our cognitive activity," she writes, "centrally involves emotional response. We discover what we think . . . partly by noticing how we feel; our investigation of our emotional geography is a major part of our search for self-knowledge."[63] Self-knowledge is indispensable to a moral life, and thus ethical conduct is impossible or fatally impaired without an investigation of feeling. The narrative ambiguities, complexities, ironies, and plural meanings so valued by scholars are more than invitations to intellectual analysis. In moments of dire conflict and inescapable choice such as Morton encounters, they make a crucial contribution to engaging the emotions of characters and of audience.

Unfortunately, bioethics hasn't begun a discussion of feeling, and the discussion won't begin until we eliminate the ancient prejudice that depicts emotion as the opposite of reason. Classical theorists in fact find occasions when emotion is a valuable ally in moral knowledge and conduct.[64] For centuries, however, metaphors deeply imbued with sexual politics have depicted reason as manly and emotion as feminine, with women defined as inherently unstable and prone to hysterical excess, as if reason didn't regularly fly off the handle. Neuroscientist Antonio R. Damasio offers one antidote to this common devaluation of feeling when he describes a man with a localized brain injury that impaired the ability to experience emotion, leaving intact the ability to reason. The man's dilemma, Damasio writes, was a capacity to know but not to feel. Significantly, this emotionless reasoner performed well on tests of moral judgment but had wholly lost the power to make decisions. Like self-knowledge, choice is clearly a prerequisite of moral action, and thus it matters greatly to the practice of ethics that decision-making appears impaired or impossible in the absence of emotion.

From a neurological as well as an ethical perspective, it makes no sense to talk of emotion and reason as opposites. Rather, according to Damasio, "certain aspects of the process of emotion and feeling are indispensable for rationality."[65] In its failures to understand the links among emotion, thought, and action, bioethics has committed itself to a stunted, calculating parody of reason that risks total paralysis or interminable hesitation in dilemmas where strong arguments compete and where principles clash. Rationality minus emotion does not account for all the relevant information. After all, the delegates of the Massachusetts Medical Society invoked a fine reason and solid principle for requiring Morton's young patient to undergo a leg amputation without anesthesia. A narrative bioethics would look beyond a calculus of principle and reason. It would require us to account for the emotion so crucial to ethical action and to the ways in which stories work on us.

The ethical implications of emotion in *The Great Moment* come into sharper focus when viewed through the work of the late Lithuanian-born French philosopher Emmanuel Levinas. Ethics for Levinas is not a rationalist enterprise deduced from higher principles or erected on an unshakable ground of theory but rather, as he puts it, ethics is first philosophy. Ethics is where philosophy begins. Further, ethics for Levinas begins with otherness—a concept he employs to designate the inherent, ineradicable, inexhaustible differences that make humans finally irreducible to a knowledge that summarizes or "contains" them. What returns us to *The Great Moment* is Levinas's famous representation of otherness in the figure or metaphor of the human face. Face as a philosophical concept far exceeds its material base in our physical features. It is not primarily a visual object. Nor is it fully knowable or containable as an object of thought. Face for Levinas evokes the "uncontainable" presence of the other person: a presence that makes an immediate ethical claim upon us. As he puts it: "The epiphany of the face is ethical."[66] The face, like narrative, exerts a kind of "call." It connects us to another person in an ethics that precedes reason, thought, and principle, an ethics born of immediate contact, akin to what takes place between Morton and his vulnerable young patient.

The face for Levinas stands for the ethical bond created in the immediate contact between two individuals that occurs primarily (although not exclusively) face-to-face. In carefully chosen words, Levinas describes the impact of the other person as an "obsession" or "shuddering" (*frémissement*), as if to indicate how far the encounter with the other taps into emotional strata more primal than logic, principle, or philosophy.[67] This prerational, impassioned, obsessive relation—the call of the other—seems clearly at play in *The Great Moment* when Morton gazes into the girl's face. The obsession or shudder of face-to-face contact is not an end-point for Levinas, however, but initiates a move into language. "Face and discourse are tied," he explains. "The face speaks. It speaks, it is in this that it renders possible and begins all discourse."[68] The face makes possible an exchange in which response—to cite a Levinasian pun—is a sign and acknowledgment of ethical responsibility. He insists: "The face opens the primordial discourse whose first word is obligation."[69] Hostage, stranger, exile: these repeated metaphors that Levinas employs to characterize the other embody a vulnerability that calls forth a responsive concern. Morton does not merely gaze into the girl's face. He speaks to her ("Are you the girl, the girl for the operation?"), and her response calls him deeper into concern. The emotion implicit in their contact—emotion that Sturges signals with a full orchestral score—is not the opposite of reason, not some trite, frenzied juice squeezed out of the limbic system. *The Great Moment* shows how emotion, speech, and obligation coalesce in an immediate contact with the other that Levinas calls, in a favorite phrase, "straightaway ethical."[70]

A straightaway ethics may be at best an ethics of right moments, when emotion inspires an inexorable drive toward moral conduct that principles alone cannot provoke. Suddenly, born of his direct contact with the young girl, Morton's doubts and conflict melt away in an immediate acceptance of a personal responsibility: an obligation that he had previously failed to acknowledge or understand. Sturges's narrative, in turn, holds the possibility of calling forth an equally responsive, straightaway ethics in the viewer. It is possible, of course, that some postmodern viewers will prefer to read Morton's heroism against the grain, alert to the dialectic by which male displays of power and virtue so regularly depend on displays of female weakness and vulnerability. Different cultures also provide different educations in pain. Norman Cousins called Americans "probably the most pain-conscious people on the face of the earth."[71] More stoical cultures might interpret the girl's approaching pain as an occasion to exercise the virtues of endurance and fortitude. With respect for cultural differences and for the conflict of interpretations, however, I cannot imagine an audience that would accept a conclusion in which Morton gazes at the girl, shrugs helplessly, and strolls unconcerned away. The film seems to require an ending consistent with an ethics of obligation. Sturges crafts a narrative whereby—short of self-betrayal or a perverse fall into evil—it is impossible for Morton *not* to do the right thing.

V. CONCLUSION: BIOETHICS MODERN AND POSTMODERN

Levinas will not resolve all the difficult questions surrounding postmodern illness. *The Great Moment* speaks to a World War II audience prepared to value self-sacrifice, duty, and the quasi-religious light that floods the final scene. It portrays a young patient who has no name or history (reduced almost to a chess piece in the game of virtue). Most important, it is a modernist work that represents ethical conduct as a matter of individual action with theological overtones. A postmodern version of the final scene would likely subtract the Ave Maria while adding a hospital attorney, a team of specialists, a drug rep, insurance providers, family, and a publisher waving a book contract. Any decisions risking legal action would entail consultation with administrators and hospital committees. Controversial action could trigger review by licensing boards. Bioethics in a postmodern world cannot avoid issues raised by the presence of vast bureaucracies and impersonal medical rationing systems.[72] It cannot ignore international issues of social justice. Does the morphine prescribed for a wealthy patient in San Diego add an unseen portion of pain to a poor patient deprived of morphine in Zaire? Who is entitled ethically—not just economically or politically—to the expensive, life-extending combination of AIDS drugs? Morton's dilemma belongs to a context different from the world of postmodern illness.

The postmodern context of institutionalized and internationalized health care is, however, precisely what lends added power to a Levinasian approach that emphasizes the value of a face-to-face straightaway ethics. Institutions often cultivate, as to their advantage, the moral twilight that ensues when they devalue individual narratives and emotional knowledge. *The Great Moment* draws attention not only to the postmodern neglect of individual faces but also to a built-in facelessness engineered to erase or obscure personal responsibility and corporate obligation. The continuity of care that once linked patients with a single doctor responsible for their medical treatment is eroded daily. Patients often no longer know who their doctor is among the convoy of specialists, team members, and rotating staff. The lack of face-to-face contact between physician and patient has ethical consequences. A narrative ethics that leans on Levinas offers to help us imagine moral values and ethical responses appropriate to a postmodern era of absent or disappearing faces.

Narrative is often indispensable in helping us grasp what our deepest values are. Some values emerge only through the twists of a particular life story. Sturges certainly makes Morton's recognition and choice of values easier by casting the patient as an attractive, helpless girl—victim and virgin—rather than a grizzled, foul-smelling vagrant. Melodrama and sentiment, however, have a complex history of engaging emotion in the affirmation of shared values, with sometimes powerful results.[73] *Uncle Tom's Cabin* proved more decisive than Abolitionist tracts in moving public opinion because it engaged emotional values attached to a specific narrative of slavery. Principles are not self-explanatory. Although the principles of nonmaleficence or beneficence might have offered Morton a reason-based shortcut to his ultimate decision, he nonetheless hesitated to act, and, as we have seen, principles led members of the Massachusetts Medical Society to an opposite decision. The principle of patient autonomy means different things to first-generation Korean Americans in Los Angeles than it means to the city's whites and blacks, but it took a team of ethnographers conducting face-to-face interviews (in effect, narrative investigations) to determine what those different meanings are and how they motivate conduct.[74] In contrast to principle alone, narrative in its detailed, emotion-rich representation of experience can help us recognize implicit values and negotiate conflicts of moral action within a new postmodern landscape of corporations, governments, and health care systems.

The Great Moment offers a timely intervention in postmodern bioethics not least because it shows that our finest achievements may come precisely when and where we least expect them: in the hallway, not at the podium. It suggests the need for an ethics attentive to everyday encounters and responsive to values submerged in the personal experience of illness.[75] It reminds us that hospital committees and regulatory boards, like other bureaucratic bodies, consist of individuals who make moral choices even while claiming to make value-free or merely financial decisions. The Great Moment does not endorse an all-out embrace of feeling that reassigns to emotion the absolutist power wrongly claimed by reason. It suggests that reason and emotion may share integrated, complementary roles in the creation of moral knowledge and ethical action. Most ethical decisions do not choose good over evil but rather, often unknowingly, honor one value or story at the expense of values and stories deemed less urgent. The unacknowledged narratives inseparable from our personal identities may matter as much as principles in our everyday moral acts. The goal of narrative bioethics is to get the stories into the open, where we can examine their values, sift their conflicts, and explore their power to work on us. I don't know about others, but the conclusion to The Great Moment—with its sentimental, melodramatic, face-to-face encounter—makes me keep wanting to replace myself.

NOTES

1. Arthur W. Frank, *The Wounded Storyteller: Body, Illness, and Ethics* (Chicago: University of Chicago Press, 1995), 23–25.
2. Keith H. Basso, *Wisdom Sits in Places: Landscape and Language among the Western Apache* (Albuquerque: University of New Mexico Press, 1996), 59.
3. Jean-François Lyotard and Jean-Loup Thébaud, *Just Gaming*, trans. Wlad Godzich (Minneapolis: University of Minnesota Press, 1985), 32–35. (Originally published in 1979.)
4. Robert Coles, *The Call of Stories: Teaching and the Moral Imagination* (Boston: Houghton Mifflin, 1989).
5. See Iris Murdoch, *The Sovereignty of Good* (New York: Schocken Books, 1971); William J. Ellos, *Narrative Ethics* (Avebury: Ashgate Publishing, 1994); and Adam Zachary Newton, *Narrative Ethics* (Cambridge, MA: Harvard University Press, 1995).
6. E. L. Doctorow, "False Documents," in *E. L. Doctorow: Essays and Conversations*, ed. Richard Trenner (Princeton: Ontario Review Press, 1983), 25, 26. (Essay originally published in 1977).
7. Elaine Scarry's justly praised book *The Body in Pain: The Making and Unmaking of the World* (New York: Oxford University Press, 1985) is not concerned with medicine or with crucial medical differences between acute pain and chronic pain. Readers tend to emphasize her opening discussion, in which torture erases or unravels conscious

world-making and thus illustrates the supposedly private and incommunicable quality of pain. This emphasis, however, slights two key points: (1) her larger argument concerns the *interpersonal* effects of torture on both torturer and tortured, and (2) her later chapters show how pain and its anticipation underwrite public, cultural, and highly communicable acts. For additional accounts, see David B. Morris, *The Culture of Pain* (Berkeley: University of California Press, 1991); Roselyne Rey, *The History of Pain*, trans. Louise Elliott Wallace, J. A. Cadden, and S. W. Cadden (Cambridge, MA: Harvard University Press, 1995); and Nigel Spivey, *Enduring Creation: Art, Pain, and Fortitude* (Berkeley: University of California Press, 2001).

8. See Isabelle Baszanger, *Inventing Pain Medicine: From the Laboratory to the Clinic*, trans. Philippa Crutchley Wallis and Monica Casper (New Brunswick, NJ: Rutgers University Press, 1998). For clinical approaches, see Ronald Melzack and Patrick D. Wall, eds., *Textbook of Pain*, 4th ed. (Edinburgh: Churchill Livingstone, 1994); for a popular account by a distinguished pain specialist, see Patrick Wall, *Pain: The Science of Suffering* (London: Weidenfeld and Nicholson, 1999).

9. In Harold Merskey and Nikolai Bogduk, eds., *Classification of Chronic Pain: Descriptions of Chronic Pain Syndromes and Definitions of Pain Terms* (Seattle: IASP Press, 1994), 210. The IASP definition was first published in 1979.

10. Timothy L. Bayer, Paul E. Baer, and Charles Early, "Situational and Psychophysiological Factors in Psychologically Induced Pain," *Pain* 44 (1991): 45–50.

11. Mark D. Sullivan, "Pain as Emotion," *Pain Forum* 5 (1996): 208–9.

12. In Merskey and Bogduk, *Classification of Chronic Pain*, 210.

13. Principlism in bioethics got its bible in Tom L. Beauchamp and James F. Childress, *Principles of Biomedical Ethics* (New York: Oxford University Press, 1979). The exchanges have been lively ever since. H. Tristram Englehardt, Jr., in *The Foundations of Bioethics* (New York: Oxford University Press, 1986), observed the impossibility, given cultural differences, of affirming any universalist "appeal to general rational justifications" (p. 14). In its second edition (1996), *Foundations* cites a well-known essay by K. Danner Clouser and Bernard Gert entitled "A Critique of Principlism" (*Journal of Medicine and Philosophy* 15 [1990]: 219–36), and in the fourth edition of *Principles of Biomedical Ethics* (1994) Beauchamp and Childress add a section ("The Place of Principles, Common Morality") in which they assert: "We defend what has sometimes been called the *four-principles approach* to biomedical ethics, and also called, somewhat disparagingly, *principlism.*" "These principles," they continue, "initially derive from considered judgments in the common morality and medical tradition" (p. 37). Significantly absent here is any claim that principles hold absolutist status or rest upon objective, universal ground. No matter how construed, principles and foundations are nonetheless a mainstay of bioethics, and reason is their pole star.

14. Mark Johnson, *Moral Imagination: Implications of Cognitive Science for Ethics* (Chicago: University of Chicago Press, 1993), 105.

15. On narrative in bioethics, see Anne Hudson Jones, "Literature and Medicine: Narrative Ethics," *The Lancet* 349 (1997): 1243–46; and "Narrative in Medical Ethics," *British Medical Journal* 318 (1999): 253–56. See also Hilde Lindemann Nelson, ed., *Stories and Their Limits: Narrative Approaches to Bioethics* (New York: Routledge, 1997).

16. David B. Morris, *Illness and Culture in the Postmodern Age* (Berkeley: University of California Press, 1998), 50–77.

17. George W. Engel, "The Need for a New Medical Model: A Challenge for Biomedicine," *Science* 196 (1977): 129–36.

18. Charles Jencks, *What Is Post-Modernism?* 2nd ed. (New York: St. Martin's Press, 1987), 14.

19. David M. Eisenberg et al., "Unconventional Medicine in the United States: Prevalence, Costs, and Patterns of Use," *New England Journal of Medicine* 328 (1993): 246–52.

20. Lori Arviso Alvord and Elizabeth Cohen Van Pelt, *The Scalpel and the Silver Bear* (New York: Bantam Books, 1999).

21. James R. Knickman and Kenneth E. Thorpe, "Financing for Healthcare," in *Jonas's Health Care Delivery in the United States*, ed. Anthony R. Kovner et al., 5th ed. (New York: Springer Publishing Company, 1995), 267–93.

22. John D. Loeser, "What Is Chronic Pain?" *Theoretical Medicine* 12 (1991): 215, 216.

23. Rolf-Detlef Treede et al., "The Cortical Representation of Pain," *Pain* 79 (1999): 105–11. On a cortical/subcortical "neuromatrix," see Ronald Melzack, "Gate Control Theory: On the Evolution of Pain Concepts," *Pain Forum* 5 (1996): 128–38. On consciousness, see Burkhart Bromm, "Consciousness, Pain, and Cortical Activity," in *Pain and the Brain: From Nociception to Cognition*, ed. Burkhart Bromm and John D. Desmeldt (New York: Raven Press, 1995), 35–59; and C. Richard Chapman and Yoshio Nakamura, "Pain and Consciousness: A Constructivist Approach," *Pain Forum* 8 (1999): 113–23. For a comprehensive approach, see Donald D. Price, *Psychological Mechanisms of Pain and Analgesia* (Seattle: IASP Press, 1999).

24. Maryann S. Bates, W. Thomas Edwards, and Karen O. Anderson, "Ethnocultural Influences on Variation in Chronic Pain Perception," *Pain* 52 (1993): 101–12; and Maryann S. Bates, *Biocultural Dimensions of Chronic Pain: Implications for Treatment of Multi-Ethnic Populations* (Albany: State University of New York Press, 1996).

25. Anita M. Unruh, "Gender Variations in Clinical Pain Experience," *Pain* 65 (1996): 123–67; and Roger B. Fillingim, ed., *Sex, Gender, and Pain* (Seattle: IASP Press, 2000).

26. Steven F. Brena, Steven H. Sanders, and Hiroshi Motoyama, "American and Japanese Chronic Low Back Pain Patients: Cross-Cultural Similarities and Differences," *The Clinical Journal of Pain* 6 (1990): 118–24.

27. See Mary-Jo DelVecchio Good et al., eds., *Pain as Human Experience: An Anthropological Perspective* (Berkeley: University of California Press, 1992); and Rod Moore and Inger Brødsgaard, "Cross-Cultural Investigations of Pain," in *Epidemiology of Pain*, ed. Iain Crombie et al. (Seattle: IASP Press, 1999), 53–80.

28. See Howard Brody, *Stories of Sickness* (New Haven: Yale University Press, 1987); Arthur Kleinman, *The Illness Narratives: Suffering, Healing, and the Human Condition* (New York: Basic Books, 1988); Anne Hunsaker Hawkins, *Reconstructing Illness: Studies in Pathography*, 2nd ed. (West Lafayette, IN: Purdue University Press, 1999); and Howard Waitzkin and Holly Magaña, "The Black Box in Somatization: Unexplained Physical Symptoms, Culture, and Narratives of Trauma," *Social Science and Medicine* 45 (1997): 811–25.

29. Kathryn Montgomery Hunter, *Doctors' Stories: The Narrative Structure of Medical Knowledge* (Princeton: Princeton University Press, 1991).

30. Trisha Greenhalgh and Brian Hurwitz, eds., *Narrative Based Medicine: Dialogue and Discourse in Clinical Practice* (London: BMJ Books, 1998).

31. James W. Pennebaker and Sandra K. Beall, "Confronting a Traumatic Event: Toward an Understanding of Inhibition and Disease," *Journal of Abnormal Psychology* 95 (1986): 274–81. See also James W. Pennebaker, "Telling Stories: The Health Benefits of Narrative," *Literature and Medicine* 19 (2000): 3–18; and Joshua M. Smyth et al., "Effects of Writing about Stressful Experiences on Symptom Reduction in Patients

with Asthma or Rheumatoid Arthritis: A Randomized Trial," *JAMA* 281 (1999): 1304–9.

32. Judith Perkins, *The Suffering Self: Pain and Narrative Representation in the Early Christian Era* (London: Routledge, 1995).

33. Mark D. Sullivan, "Between First-person and Third-person Accounts of Pain in Clinical Medicine," paper delivered at the 9th World Congress on Pain, Vienna, 1999.

34. See, among others, David A. Williams and Beverly E. Thorn, "An Empirical Assessment of Pain Beliefs," *Pain* 36 (1989): 351–58; David A. Williams and Francis J. Keefe, "Pain Beliefs and the Use of Cognitive-Behavioral Coping Strategies," *Pain* 46 (1991): 185–90; Mark P. Jensen and Paul Karoly, "Pain-Specific Beliefs, Perceived Symptom Severity, and Adjustment to Chronic Pain," *The Clinical Journal of Pain* 8, no. 2 (1992): 123–30; and David A. Williams, Michael E. Robinson, and Michael E. Geisser, "Pain Beliefs: Assessment and Utility," *Pain* 59 (1994): 71–78.

35. Douglas E. DeGood and Michael S. Shutty, Jr., "Assessment of Pain Beliefs, Coping, and Self-Efficacy," in *Handbook of Pain Assessment*, ed. Dennis C. Turk and Ronald Melzack (New York: Guilford Press, 1992), 214–34.

36. See Ranjan Roy, *The Social Context of the Chronic Pain Sufferer* (Toronto: University of Toronto Press, 1992); and Robert J. Gatchel and Dennis C. Turk, eds., *Psychosocial Factors in Pain: Critical Perspectives* (New York: Guilford Press, 1999).

37. Stanley J. Bigos et al., "A Prospective Study of Work Perceptions and Psychosocial Factors Affecting the Report of Back Injury," *Spine* 16 (1991): 1–6.

38. Jay D. Summers et al., "Psychosocial Factors in Chronic Spinal Cord Injury Pain," *Pain* 47 (1991): 183–89.

39. In addition to works cited earlier, see Tod Chambers, *The Fiction of Bioethics: Cases as Literary Texts* (New York: Routledge, 1999); Sally Gadow, "Relational Narrative: The Postmodern Turn in Nursing Ethics," *Scholarly Inquiry for Nursing Practice: An International Journal* 13 (1999): 57–70; and Kathryn Montgomery, "Literature, Literary Studies, and Medical Ethics: The Interdisciplinary Question," *Hastings Center Report* 31, no. 3 (2001): 36–43.

40. Alasdair MacIntyre, *After Virtue: A Study in Moral Theory* (Notre Dame, IN: Notre Dame University Press, 1981), 201, 197.

41. Harald Schrader et al., "Natural Evolution of Late Whiplash Syndrome outside the Mediocolegal Context," *The Lancet* 347 (1996): 1207–11. See also Bogdan P. Radanov et al., "Course of Psychological Variables in Whiplash Injury: A Two-Year Follow-up with Age, Gender, and Education Pair-Matched Patients," *Pain* 64 (1996): 429–34.

42. Wilbert E. Fordyce, ed., *Back Pain in the Workplace: Management of Disability in Nonspecific Conditions* (Seattle: IASP Press, 1995), xiii.

43. George Mendelson, "Compensation and Chronic Pain," *Pain* 48 (1992): 121–23.

44. My account is based on Robert Pear, "Mothers on Medicaid Overcharged for Pain Relief," *New York Times*, March 8, 1999.

45. Quotations related to the case of Mrs. Chavez come from the *New York Times* report by Robert Pear (note 44).

46. Pierre Macherey, *A Theory of Literary Production*, trans. Geoffrey Wall (London: Routledge and Kegan Paul, 1978), 77–78. (Essay originally published in 1966).

47. John K. Ingelhart, "The American Health Care System: Expenditures," *New England Journal of Medicine* 340 (1999): 70–76.

48. SUPPORT Principal Investigators, "A Controlled Trial to Improve Care for Seriously Ill Hospitalized Patients," *JAMA* 274 (1995): 1591–98.

49. "Undertreatment of acute pain and chronic cancer pain persists despite decades of efforts to provide clinicians with information about analgesics" (American Pain Society Quality of Care Committee, "Quality Improvement Guidelines for the Treatment of Acute Pain and Cancer Pain," *JAMA* 274 [1995]: 1874).

50. J. Stephenson, "Experts Say AIDS Pain 'Dramatically Undertreated,'" *JAMA* 276 (1996): 1369–70.

51. C. Stratton Hill, Jr., "The Negative Influence of Licensing and Disciplinary Boards and Drug Enforcement Agencies on Pain Treatment with Opioid Analgesics," *Journal of Pharmaceutical Care in Pain and Symptom Control* 1 (1993): 43–62.

52. In 1989, pioneering pain specialist John Bonica declared that "no medical school has a pain curriculum" (quoted in Richard Weiner, "An Interview with John J. Bonica, M.D.," *Pain Practitioner* 1 [1989]: 2). A 1988 study of British medical schools found that four had no instruction about pain while the others averaged a mere three hours over five years (D. Marcer and S. Deighton, "Intractable Pain: A Neglected Area of Medical Education in the UK," *Journal of the Royal Society of Medicine* 81 [1988]: 689–700). In acknowledgment of such deficiencies, the International Association for the Study of Pain published *Core Curriculum for Professional Education in Pain,* ed. Howard L. Fields (Seattle: IASP Press, 1989), with a second edition appearing in 1995.

53. "Patients know that their conduct in seeking various avenues to achieve pain relief is often stereotyped as 'drug-seeking behavior' by some care providers" (Samir K. Ballas, *Sickle Cell Pain* [Seattle: IASP Press, 1998], 287).

54. R. Sean Morrison et al., "'We Don't Carry That': Failure of Pharmacies in Predominantly Nonwhite Neighborhoods to Stock Opioid Analgesics," *New England Journal of Medicine* 342 (2000): 1023–26.

55. Anthony DePalma, "For Mexicans, Pain Relief Is Both a Medical and a Political Problem," *New York Times,* June 19, 1996.

56. Ben A. Rich, "A Legacy of Shame: Bioethics and the Culture of Pain," *Journal of Medical Humanities* 18 (1997): 233–59.

57. In addition to Morris's *The Culture of Pain* and Spivey's *Enduring Creation,* see Esther Cohen, "The Animated Pain of the Body," *American Historical Review* 18 (2000): 36–65.

58. See, among others, Daniel P. Goleman, *Emotional Intelligence: Why It Can Matter More Than IQ for Character, Health, and Lifelong Achievement* (New York: Bantam Books, 1995); Megan Boler, *Feeling Power: Emotions and Education* (New York: Routledge, 1999); and Nancy J. Chodorow, *The Power of Feelings: Personal Meaning in Psychoanalysis, Gender, and Culture* (New Haven: Yale University Press, 1999).

59. Ellen Singer More and Maureen A. Milligan, eds., *The Empathic Practitioner: Empathy, Gender, and Medicine* (New Brunswick, NJ: Rutgers University Press, 1994).

60. *The Great Moment* is on videocassette (MCA Universal #81022). The screenplay, entitled *Triumph over Pain,* is available in *Four More Screenplays by Preston Sturges,* introduction by Brian Henderson (Berkeley: University of California Press, 1995). Paramount abridged and reedited Sturges's film before releasing it, so the film is not identical with the screenplay, which is based on material in René Fülöp-Miller's *Triumph over Pain: The Story of Anesthesia,* trans. Eden and Cedar Paul (New York: Literary Guild of America, 1938).

61. Edmund D. Pellegrino, "Emerging Ethical Issues in Palliative Care," *JAMA* 279 (1998): 1521–22.

62. Rafael Campo, *The Desire to Heal: A Doctor's Education in Empathy, Identity, and Poetry* (New York: Norton, 1997), 132. First published as *The Poetry of Healing: A Doctor's Education in Empathy, Identity, and Desire.*

63. Martha C. Nussbaum, *The Fragility of Goodness: Luck and Ethics in Greek Tragedy and Philosophy* (Cambridge: Cambridge University Press, 1986), 15.

64. Classical concepts of emotion, while aware of its potential danger and irrationalism, also see occasions when it is indispensable to moral knowledge and action. See, for example, John M. Cooper, *Reason and Emotion: Essays on Ancient Moral Psychology and Ethical Theory* (Princeton: Princeton University Press, 1999); and Diana Fritz Cates, *Choosing to Feel: Virtue, Friendship, and Compassion for Friends* (Notre Dame, IN: Notre Dame University Press, 1997).

65. Antonio R. Damasio, *Descartes's Error: Emotion, Reason, and the Human Brain* (New York: Avon Books, 1994), xiii.

66. Emmanuel Levinas, *Totality and Infinity: An Essay on Exteriority*, trans. Alphonso Lingis (Pittsburgh: Duquesne University Press, 1969), 199 (III.B.2). For commentary, see Richard A. Cohen, ed., *Face to Face with Levinas* (Albany: State University of New York Press, 1986); Robert Bernasconi and Simon Critchley, eds., *Re-Reading Levinas* (Bloomington: Indiana University Press, 1991); and Jacques Derrida, *Adieu to Emmanuel Levinas*, trans. Pascale-Anne Brault and Michael Naas (Stanford: Stanford University Press, 1999). (Essay originally published in 1997). My aim is not to offer a critique of Levinas—questioning whether "face" serves much like the a priori standards he rejects or whether he deals adequately with issues of social justice—but to explore application of his impressive main concepts.

67. "The neighbor assigns me before I designate him. This is a modality not of a knowing, but of an obsession, a shuddering of the human quite different from cognition" (Emmanuel Levinas, *Otherwise Than Being or Beyond Essence*, trans. Alphonso Lingis [Pittsburgh: Duquesne University Press, 1981], 87). Levinas's note to this passage (p. 192) says that "shuddering" translates the Platonic term *phrike* from *Phaedrus*, which is the dialogue where Socrates calls love a divine madness that lifts the soul toward truth.

68. Emmanuel Levinas, *Ethics and Infinity: Conversations with Philippe Nemo*, trans. Richard A. Cohen (Pittsburgh: Duquesne University Press, 1985), 87.

69. Levinas, *Totality and Infinity*, 201.

70. Levinas, *Ethics and Infinity*, 85, 87 ("d'emblée éthique").

71. Norman Cousins, *Anatomy of an Illness as Perceived by the Patient: Reflections on Healing and Regeneration* (New York: Norton, 1979), 89.

72. See Robert B. Baker et al., eds., *The American Medical Ethics Revolution: How the AMA's Code of Ethics Has Transformed Physicians' Relationships to Patients, Professionals, and Society* (Baltimore: Johns Hopkins University Press, 1999); and David A. Bennahum, ed., *Managed Care: Financial, Legal, and Ethical Issues* (Cleveland: Pilgrim Press, 1999).

73. Jane P. Tompkins, *Sentimental Designs: The Cultural Work of American Fiction, 1790–1860* (New York: Oxford University Press, 1985).

74. Leslie A. Blackhall et al., "Ethnicity and Attitudes toward Patient Autonomy," *JAMA* 274 (1995): 820–25.

75. Arthur W. Frank, "First-person Microethics: Deriving Principles from Below," *Hastings Center Report* 28, no. 4 (1998): 37–42; and Morris, *Illness and Culture*, 259–69.

CHAPTER 21

THE STORY INSIDE
JOANNE TRAUTMANN BANKS

N arrative inevitably expresses and transforms who we are at every level of our being: the organic, the symbolic, the social, and the spiritual. This is an immodest claim, I know, but I am only making explicit what each of the other writers in this collection has assumed. I will try to show that stories in all their forms satisfy our deepest selves; that far from being an amusement or an aesthetic patina on our daily lives, narrative is fundamental to our bodies, minds, communities, and souls. It follows that bringing a full understanding of narrative to our work as ethicists changes all our thoughts, all our actions. The narrative urge is central, although occasionally perilous, even in that complicated form of self and other enacted in bioethics practice.

THE ORGANIC

At the *organic* level, for instance, our bodies give birth to certain narrative ways of perceiving the world. Because our eyes are located in the front of our heads, we usually move forward instead of sidling back and forth like the stem-eyed crab or waving our limbs about like the stationary sea anemone. As a consequence of human motion, we tend to believe in the inherent rightness of plot. That is, we believe with our organic selves in narrative, whose basic delight is, "Go forward, turn the page, to discover what happens next." Seen from this angle, walking is itself a type of plot line.

Of course, writers have also created radical, experimental narratives that might in this context be called crab or anemone stories. They don't move forward in the traditional way but are nonetheless born of our cells. Virginia Woolf's short prose piece "Kew Gardens" is a good example of an anemone story in which, from a snail's perspective, flowers, insects, and people seem to undulate in an "irregular and aimless movement."[1] Viewed as a whole, however, "Kew Gardens" has a purpose—call it the demonstration of pleasing aesthetic patterns in the natural world from insect to human—just as the fluttering cilia on our cells purposively move fluids over cellular surfaces. Or consider the crablike movement of Kurosawa's famous cinematic narrative *Rashomon*:[2] four people involved in a rape-murder tell four different sides of the story, each one an attempt to move the others toward the "right" version. It seems to me that this kind of narrative is similar to the oscillatory movement that directs our bodies toward homeostasis. On the basis of our feedback and control systems, elements in the body go from one side to another in an attempt to find the balance we need. In fact, the eminent philosopher of religion Paul Tillich finds this kind of mechanism on each of the levels of life with which I am concerned.[3] We open and close around data, open and close, until we die. Thus, we never stay in the homeostatic condition for very long; no sooner does the body (likewise, the symbolic, social, and spiritual self) settle into a situation than a stimulus comes along to push for change—just as, in *Rashomon*, the final version remains forever elusive.

In this way, various parts of our bodies express elements of narrative. But sometimes our whole bodies are swept up into one grand drama. When we burst into a belly laugh, for instance, or when we are pushed over the top into orgasm, our bodies become for an instant a story of pleasure that is congruous with our existence. And likewise when we are desperately ill, our bodies may strike us as, simultaneously, theater, cast, and plot; our lives, as runaway organicity. Glucose and insulin face off in a duel on one patient's bloody stage, and heroic T-cells chase down villainous microbes on another's. Even severely retarded persons with minimal language skills or people left comatose by strokes tell their stories by way of their physical presences.[4] It becomes the job of the narrative ethicist, therefore, to interpret these corporeal events as a literary critic would a Shakespearean play.

If narrative thus *expresses* our biological selves, does it also *transform* our bodies, as I have said in the sweeping sentence with which this argument begins? At this stage of our knowledge, I can only suspect so. Some testimony comes from sociologist Arthur Frank, who speaks from profound personal experience of illness when he declares, "Bodies are realized—not just represented but created—in the stories they tell."[5] As if to demonstrate that point, the renowned Russian physician A. R. Luria presents the case of a brain-damaged patient who reconstructs himself by keeping a fragmented diary that gradually attains a narrative form.[6] Contemporary neuroscientists are beginning to show precisely how such a thing can happen. After decades of believing that nothing can replace brain cells, once destroyed, scientists are using the new, sophisticated imaging techniques (nuclear magnetic resonance [NMR] scans and positron emission tomography [PET] scans) to reveal the exciting news that experience causes our brains to be reorganized. A growing group of scientists believes that behavior not only changes our personhood as understood broadly—this has long been axiomatic—but, more specifically, that behavior is the principal determinant of alterations in our nervous system. First in animals, then in physically compromised humans, and finally in healthy people, studies have detailed the changes consequent to experience.[7] This research makes it likely that reading and telling and listening to stories— indeed forms of experience—have affected our bodies for millennia. It is also entirely possible that new forms of stories—for example, computer-generated, community-narrated stories—will become part of our brains and therefore our-selves in ways that only the passing of more millennia will make clear.

THE SYMBOLIC

When we operate on the *symbolic* level, no such speculation is required. It is clear that human beings create symbols and are, in turn, transformed by them. Although there is an old debate about the chronological relation of language to thinking, most people believe that symbols develop shortly after language does. (Language is itself symbolic, of course, in that it only *represents* reality and is not the concrete thing itself.) Therefore, small children already have some ideas about such common symbols as a red traffic light and the American flag. Older children and adults are very nearly awash in the effects of symbolism, for good or ill. That's because symbols seldom appear without their attendant narratives. In this respect, a symbol is like a molecule—say, H_2O—in which the oxygen atom has two sites into which the hydrogen atoms are drawn. Just so does a symbol draw a story or, more often, a vast number of stories generated by each individual.

Take the complicated symbol "hospital." I recently went with two adolescent girls to the hospital to see their grandfather, who had just emerged from a coma. They entered two different buildings, symbolically, because "hospital" set off an elaborate horror tale for the older girl, who could barely look at her grandfather, let alone the dying man in the next bed; whereas the younger girl, who fantasizes her-self as an actress, was exhilarated by the scene and even titillated when she was thereafter introduced to a woman whose leg had just been amputated. The next time the two girls go to a hospital, whether as visitors or patients, they will surely carry this last experience with them, for symbols accrue around the self as we grow older. As adults, most of us have learned to camouflage the faces we present to soci-ety,[8] but we are no less impressionable than the two girls to symbols of our own.

Moreover, all of us with normally functioning brains are vulnerable to sym-bolic stories. According to certain cognitive psychologists who combine qualita-tive and quantitative research methods, our reception of stories is not necessarily affected by how smart we are or how little trained in critical reading and listening—though, naturally, training enables us to make far better use of our nar-rative experiences. Nor does it make any difference if the story is technically "good" or "bad," or whether or not ethics committee members are a bit sleepy on the day when a patient's story is presented to them. Richard Gerrig would say that once the members perceive the story at all, once they let it in, they will be "trans-ported" to the story's sphere of meaning and there "perform" the story to an extent of which they may even be unaware.[9] Gerrig's argument, as teachers of lit-erature have long wished to believe, is that this type of empathy with stories—however told—is an inherent human ability. I would argue that along with empathy comes a degree of responsibility for the person whose sphere of self we have entered as a guest, and therein lies the ethical component of narrative.

The stories heard and read by bioethicists are generally complicated symbolic structures. In my experience, it has proved helpful for caregivers intent on decoding such structures to learn that clinical stories can often be classified according to literary nomenclature for narrative and dramatic types. This labeling has a long history, going back at least as far as Aristotle, who initially defined tragedy and comedy, together with their transformative effects on the self.[10] Today the traditional literary genres are being soundly contested, but bioethicists need not get into the technical aspects of the scholarly debate in order to use the conventional groupings or to understand them in their common meanings. For instance, the tragic stories that are found every day along hospital and clinic corridors tend to call forth in their witnessess what classical tragedy evokes in the audience. Being present to tragedy elicits catharsis in the spectator, said Aristotle, who, as a physician's son, liked to use medical terms. That is, by being drawn into tragic stories, we are purged of strong emotions that can get in the way of honest perspectives. Ethicists and clinicians—and all of humanity, for that matter—don't want to admit into their psychological inner sanctums the full elements of tragedy, lest it seem that the world, and therefore the witnesses themselves, are out of control and liable to despair. But they thereby miss out on the cleansing benefits of tragedy and are unable to go on to the higher forms of comedy, which, as I understand them, have little to do with humor of the usual sort and much to do with continuance, community, and cathartic calmness.[11] In fact, bioethicists have been honored by society with unusual opportunities to pass *through* tragedy to a serene acceptance of life's integrity in the face of the despair and disgust that is everywhere in medicine and often within ourselves as well. These terms—*integrity, despair, disgust*—are used by psychologist Erik Erikson to describe the last stage of self-fulfillment in his famous "life cycle," during which the self has the chance to achieve "wisdom." (His widow has recently written that they had discovered a further stage, "gerotranscendence," late in their lives.[12]) My point is that in making ourselves open to medical tragedies and life's ultimate "comedies" we have the opportunity to reach our fullest, our best, identities.

Yet the majority of stories heard in bioethics are probably neither tragic nor comic in the senses in which I have been describing them. Often ethicists hear narratives that can best be described by other literary categories, such as pathos, which can be viewed as a potential tragedy that short-circuits its own possibilities and therefore elicits only temporary emotions. For examples, turn to any *Reader's Digest* story of a disabled person's overcoming great odds. Occasionally, the teller of the tale cannot resist satirizing the other narrative participants, because satire is the literary genre that bleeds off our tension, resentment, boredom, and helplessness. Bioethicists have heard, as well as enacted, a good many detective stories, too. There was a mystery, but I, the health care provider, or we, the ethics committee, have solved it. Melodrama is a genre that is particularly risky in committee contexts in that it prompts us to see ourselves in stereotypical roles, often "hero" (the clinician or ethicist), who saves the day, and "victim" (the patient). A constant of these simpler literary categories is that they engender an us-versus-them perspective, in which little significant growth of the self can occur. But all literary genres, whether grand or commonplace, serve as symbolic conveyances of universal human experiences and opportunities.

THE SOCIAL

We are also *social* beings, I have said, and on it is on this level of functioning that ethicists and ethics committee members as practitioners of narrative ethics discover their true powers. But I am obliged to ask, first, how the self can be expressed and acted upon when each unique individual is also charged with functioning as a member of the group. In committees, for example, does group expression supersede self-expression? The best answer has been given by the field theory psychologists.[13] They are the people for whom the self cannot be said to exist *except* in relation to others. For them, the self is best defined as the nexus of everything that influences us. For instance, a doctor cannot be said to be truly a doctor until he or she is interacting with a patient or a medical issue. Likewise, the ethical self is a comparatively meaningless concept until it behaves responsibly toward another.

The physician and novelist who publishes under the name of Samuel Shem has endorsed this idea of the self.[14] Shem writes that "the primary motivation of human beings is the desire for connection," and he underscores "the shift of focus [in Western thought] from the centrality of *the* [Freudian] *self* to the centrality of . . . *the self-in-relationship*" (pp. 43–44). He asserts that "the seeds of human misery are planted in disconnections, violations, isolation, and domination, and the core of healthy growth is the movement from isolation toward connection" (p. 44). These thoughts echo backwards through the twentieth century. Sigmund Freud held that a significant part of the healthy self was the ability to love (the other part was, of course, the ability to be productive and creative). To Freud we could add the names of sociologists, reader-response literary critics, philosophical phenomenologists, Jungian psychologists, novelists, and medical anthropologists.[15] One of them, James Hillman, pictures the process of mutual growth between doctor and a patient as a kind of singer's contest, a round like *Frère Jacques*, in which each singer of the tale follows closely after the other, and thereby takes responsibility for both of them.

I return to Samuel Shem for a *narrative* expression of a doctor's relationships with patients. In the following passage from "*Mount Misery*," the sequel to Shem's widely read novel *The House of God*, a physician meditates on how his work as a reader of patients' stories has enabled him to move from depression to freedom:

> I realized how much my vision had broadened. Instead of seeing just bodies, I was seeing people, reading people, sensing in people's faces and postures and words and in the intangible stuff, some truth about the person, not only in terms of each life, but in each as part of any life, of life itself. I saw the sorrow behind the smile, the years of pain pulling out the lines from the corners of the mouth and eyes, the rage provoking the

scar, the weight of nostalgia tugging down the lip, even the smile behind the sorrow. From my year of focusing on the something else besides what these people were showing me consciously, they had become more translucent yet more substantial, in the way that the translucency of a deep-sea creature reveals the bones, the guts, the feathery beat of the heart, that glassy-ribbed heart.[16]

If we assume the truth of the relational self, ethicists receive a personal dividend as they attend to one another's interpretations of the patient's story—their work contributes fundamentally to their own self-development. "These parents don't want their Down's baby to have life-saving surgery?" asks one ethics committee member. Her question suddenly provokes in her own mind an image of the sweet retarded boy who lived next door one summer when she was ten. A nurse explains why he has chosen to work in hospice care, and the joy he expresses mitigates, just a little, the ethicist's fear of her own death. Indeed, self-development is not so much work in this context as a variety of significant and serious play, for much of it goes on naturally—even unconsciously, as Gerrig has demonstrated—within the social context of shared tastes and a common search for meaning.

Granted, seeing the ethics committee as the site of memory and maturation is markedly different from our culture's view of such activities. "I want to die in the middle of a committee meeting," runs one joke, "because then the transition from life to death would be imperceptible." Witticisms do, however, point to an irritating aspect of committee work about which most of us have complained—that committees are better at talking than at getting things done. To be sure, ethics committees are set up to act, or at least to decide upon the recommendation of an action. But long talks do, and must, take place. In this respect, I value Richard Rorty's conception of the moral "conversation," as John D. Arras has presented it. Conversation "desires only its own continuation in a limitless quest for novelty. It refuses to seek a final resting place in some moral, social, or scientific bedrock."[17] Lest this unending conversation sound dangerously vague or simply exhausting, it is good to remember that we have seen this kind of continual closing and reopening in the constant readjustment of homeostasis in our organic selves. True, our symbolic selves tell and receive stories that cry out for the "sense of an ending," as critic Frank Kermode puts the matter.[18] But that completion is only a transient "sense." Far more basic to our symbolic and social worlds is the familiar phrase "to be continued."[19]

THE SPIRITUAL

Continuation is basic to much of our *spiritual* world as well. John Wesley liked to speak of "going on toward" perfection, rather than achieving it. An ancient Asian maxim runs: "The journey, not the arrival, matters." Furthermore, all major religions recognize that the spiritual dimension is not separate from the others—those I have here called the organic, symbolic, and social—and that they operate simultaneously in "multidimensional unity," as Tillich was fond of saying in the last years of his life, not in tiers from an imagined high of spirituality to a low of organicity, but simultaneously. Thus, I do not want my occasional use of "level" to imply a hierarchy of the self.

The practice of narrative ethics also speaks to our spiritual selves in ways that need have nothing to do with religion in any doctrinal sense. The doctor-poet from New Jersey, William Carlos Williams, seems to have lost his famous way with words when it came to describing the wonder that the stories of his patients had opened up for him. Tacitly admitting that the transcendental experience is ultimately inexpressible, he refers to it as "the thing": "My 'medicine' [it is fair to substitute "my work as an ethicist"] ... gained me entrance to these secret gardens of the self.... [J]ust there, the thing, in all its greatest beauty, may for a moment be freed to fly for a moment ... about the room ... instant and perfect: it comes, it is there, and it vanishes. But I have seen it, clearly. I have seen it."[20]

So have most of us who view the world through, and as, narrative. Although we don't often say it aloud, we know that there are timeless moments (Williams's moment might be one) when we give over our self to another person. Sometimes the merging with people (or something else in the natural world) goes so far that we are not even conscious of being present as a separate entity at all. James Joyce called such instances "epiphanies." Virginia Woolf called them "moments of being." Mystics say that they are unions with God. Call them what you will, but at those times we realize with full force the universal spiritual paradox that in order to gain the self, we must be willing to lose it.

NOTES

1. Virginia Woolf, "Kew Gardens," in *The Complete Shorter Fiction of Virginia Woolf* (San Diego: Harcourt, Brace, Jovanovich, 1985), 89.
2. Akira Kurosawa, *Rashomon* (Tokyo, 1950).
3. Paul Tillich, "The Meaning of Health," *Perspectives in Biology and Medicine* 5 (1961): 92–100.
4. Joanne Trautmann Banks, "Furthermore: Caring for People Who Cannot Respond," *Academic Medicine* 66 (1991): 202–3.
5. Arthur W. Frank, *The Wounded Storyteller: Body, Illness, and Ethics* (Chicago: University of Chicago Press, 1995), 52.
6. A. R. Luria, *The Man with the Shattered World: The History of a Brain Wound*, trans. L. Solotaroff (New York: Basic Books, 1972).
7. See E. I. Knudsen, "Capacity for Plasticity in the Adult Owl Auditory System Expanded by Juvenile Experience," *Science* 279 (1998): 1531–33; Elizabeth Gould et al., "Neurogenesis in the Neocortex of Adult Primates," *Science* 286 (1999): 548–52; S. Knecht et al., "Cortical Reorganization in Human Amputees and Mislocalization of Painful Stimuli to the Phantom Limb," *Neuroscience Letters* 201 (1995): 262–64; and T. Elbert et al., "Increased Cortical Representation of the Fingers of the Left Hand in String Players," *Science* 270 (1995): 305–7.

8. Erving Goffman, *The Presentation of Self in Everyday Life* (Garden City, NY: Doubleday, 1959).

9. Richard J. Gerrig, *Experiencing Narrative Worlds: On the Psychological Activities of Reading* (New Haven: Yale University Press, 1993), 2.

10. Aristotle, *Poetics*, in *Aristotle on the Art of Fiction: An English Translation of Aristotle's Poetics*, trans. L. J. Potts (Cambridge: Cambridge University Press, 1953).

11. Joanne Trautmann Banks, "Medicine and the Comic Spirit," John P. McGovern Award Lectureship of the American Osler Society, 1988.

12. Erik H. Erikson and Joan M. Erikson, *The Life Cycle Completed: Extended Version* (New York: Norton, 1997), 123–29.

13. Kurt Lewin, *Field Theory in Social Science* (New York: Harper, 1951); and Harry S. Sullivan, "Definitions," in *The Interpersonal Theory of Psychiatry*, ed. H. S. Perry and M. L. Gawel (New York: W. W. Norton, 1953), 13–30.

14. Samuel Shem, "Psychiatry and Literature: A Relational Perspective," *Literature and Medicine* 10 (1991): 42–65. Subsequent page references to this work appear in parentheses in the text.

15. Natan Sznaider, "The Sociology of Compassion: A Study in the Sociology of Morals," *Cultural Values* 2 (1998): 117–39; Elizabeth Freund, *The Return of the Reader: Reader-Response Criticism* (London: Methuen, 1987); Adam Zachary Newton, *Narrative Ethics* (Cambridge, MA: Harvard University Press, 1995); Maurice Merleau-Ponty, *The Primacy of Perception and Other Essays on Phenomenological Psychology, the Philosophy of Art, History, and Politics*, ed. J. M. Edie (Evanston, IL: Northwestern University Press, 1964); James Hillman, "The Fiction of Case History: A Round," in *Religion as Story*, ed. J. B. Wiggins (New York: Harper and Row, 1975); Virginia Woolf, *The Waves* [1931] (Oxford: Blackwell, 1993); and Arthur Kleinman, "Anthropology of Bioethics," in *Writing at the Margin: Discourse between Anthropology and Medicine* (Berkeley: University of California Press, 1995), 41–67.

16. Samuel Shem, *Mount Misery* (New York: Ballantine, 1997), 436.

17. John D. Arras, "Nice Story, but So What? Narrative and Justification in Ethics," in *Stories and Their Limits: Narative Approaches to Bioethics*, ed. Hilde Lindemann Nelson (New York: Routledge, 1997), 65–88.

18. Frank Kermode, *The Sense of an Ending: Studies in the Theory of Fiction* (Oxford: Oxford University Press, 1967).

19. L. J. Schneiderman, "Sequel: A Short Story," *Literature and Medicine* 5 (1986): 75–83.

20. William Carlos Williams, *The Autobiography of William Carlos Williams* (New York: New Directions, 1967), 288–89.

Charles M. Anderson is professor of rhetoric and writing at the University of Arkansas at Little Rock, where he teaches expository and technical writing. He also teaches medical ethics and literature and medicine at the University of Arkansas for Medical Sciences. His major publications include *Richard Selzer and the Rhetoric of Surgery* (Southern Illinois University, 1989) and an edited collection with Marian MacCurdy entitled *Writing and Healing: Toward an Informed Practice* (National Council of Teachers of English Press, 2000). He recently edited a special issue of *Literature and Medicine* (Spring 2000) focused on writing and healing. Anderson has presented at numerous conferences, including the National Council of Teachers of English, College Composition and Communication, the American College of Physicians, and the American Society for Bioethics and Humanities. He is currently completing a memoir entitled *Journey Time*, which is both the fruit and the source of his work with healing narratives over the past twenty years.

Joanne Trautmann Banks became the first full-time professor of literature at a medical school when, in 1972, she joined the faculty of Pennsylvania State University's College of Medicine. Her activities there included being Humanities Attending in a clinic as well as serving on a clinical ethics committee. She is known for her work on Virginia Woolf, having edited Woolf's *Letters.* (Harcourt, Brace, 1975–1980). She also edited *Literature and Medicine: An Annotated Bibliography* (Society for health and Human Values, 1975; University of Pittsburgh, 1981), which contains over fourteen hundred literary works that illuminate thirty-nine topics, including abortion, euthanasia, and other topics in biomedical ethics.

Wayne Booth is professor of English emeritus at the University of Chicago, where he has taught for more than forty years. Of his many works related to this book, the most significant are probably *The Rhetoric of Fiction* (University of Chicago Press, 1961, 1983) and *The Company We Keep: An Ethics of Fiction* (University of California, 1988). He is currently working on a book on how the rhetoric of the "best" scientific thinkers overlaps with the rhetoric of the "best" theologians.

Howard Brody received his M.D. and Ph.D. in philosophy from Michigan State University and completed a family practice residency at the University of Virginia. He is currently professor of family practice and philosophy and director of the Center for Ethics and Humanities in the Life Sciences at Michigan State University. He is currently preparing a revised edition of his book *Stories of Sickness* (Yale, 1987). He is also the author of *The Healer's Power* (Yale, 1992).

Jerome Bruner, born in New York in 1915, was educated at Duke and Harvard, receiving his Ph.D. in psychology from Harvard. He has taught at Harvard and Oxford, and is currently a university professor at New York University, where he is also a member of the Faculty of Law. His 1956 book, *A Study of Thinking* (Wiley, 1956), is often taken as the kick-off of the so-called cognitive revolution, psychology's turning away from behaviorism to the study of the mind. His interest in how the mind works has led him into many topics—the growth of the mind from infancy on, the shaping of mental processes by culture's ways, the reality-constructing operations of cognition, and, lately, the importance of narrative as a mode of thought and of representing the world. His most recent book is *Making Stories: Law, Literature, Life* (Farrar, Straus, and Giroux, 2002) He has been favored by many honors, including the Balzan Prize in 1987 and a doctorate *honoris causa* from Harvard in 1997.

Ronald A. Carson is the author of a monograph on Sartre and of many articles, chapters, and reviews in both humanities and medical publications, including the entry "Interpretation" in the *Encyclopedia of Bioethics* (Macmillan, 1995). He is coeditor of and contributor to several books, most recently (with Chester R. Burns and Thomas R. Cole) *Practicing the Medical Humanities: Forms of Engagement*, University Publishing Group, forthcoming. He is a founder and coeditor of the *Medical Humanities Review*, a founding member of the editorial board of the British journal *Medical Humanities*, and a contributing editor of *Literature and Medicine* and *Second Opinion*. Carson is currently Harris L. Kempner Distinguished Professor and Director of the Institute for the Medical Humanities at the University of Texas Medical Branch at Galveston.

Tod Chambers is assistant professor of medical ethics and humanities and of medicine at Northwestern University Medical School. His research interests focus on the rhetorical features in bioethics discourse and cross-cultural issues in clinical medicine. His book *The Fiction of Bioethics* (Routledge, 1999) examines the way case narratives in medical ethics rhetorically support philosophical ideas. He is presently coediting with Carl Elliott a book titled *Prozac as a Way of Life*, which will be published by the University of North Carolina Press.

Rita Charon is professor of clinical medicine and director of the Program in Narrative Medicine at the College of Physicians and Surgeons of Columbia University, where she practices general internal medicine and teaches literature, internal medicine, and ethics. She has written and lectured extensively on literature and medicine, empathy, narrative ethics, and the novels of Henry James. She is editor in chief, along with Professor Maura Spiegel, of *Literature and Medicine.* She is now working on a book called *Narrative Medicine.*

Marcia Day Childress holds a Ph.D. in English literature from the University of Virginia. She is associate professor of medical education and codirector of the University of Virginia's School of Medicine's Program of Humanities in Medicine. She codirects the Medical Center Hour, the School of Medicine's weekly forum fostering conversation between medicine and society on current health-related issues and controversies. In addition, she is co–principal investigator on the University of Virginia's curriculum development grants in spirituality and medicine. She serves on the hospital ethics committee and the University of Virginia Faculty Senate and is involved in university-wide initiatives concerning women and diversity. She has published articles in *Academic Medicine, Literature and Medicine, Second Opinion,* and *The Pharos.*

Larry R. Churchill is professor and former chair of the Department of Social Medicine in the School of Medicine, the University of North Carolina at Chapel Hill. His current research focuses on the ethics of managed care, justice in health policy, research with human subjects, and ethical issues around care at the end of life. Churchill is the author or editor of seven books and numerous essays, articles, and book chapters. He is also coeditor of *Studies in Social Medicine,* a series with the University of North Carolina Press. Churchill is codirector of the newly formed Center for Health Ethics and Policy at the University of North Carolina, a research and education unit that focuses on the ethical questions of health policy in genomics/genetics, end of life care, and access to medical services. As of July 2002, he will be the Anne Geddes Stohlman Professor of Medical Ethics, Vanderbilt University.

Julia E. Connelly is professor of medicine and codirector of the Program of the Humanities in Medicine at the University of Virginia School of Medicine, where she has been a faculty member since 1983. In her clinical work, she specializes in primary care internal medicine and medical psychiatry. She works in a medical office in the rural community of Orange, Virginia. Since 1990, she has been medical director of the Orange County Nursing Home. In 1994, she was president of the Society for Health and Human Values (now the American Society for Bioethics and Humanities). She has published stories and essays that reflect her interest in medicine and the humanities; the focus of much of her work is on the nature of the patient-physician relationship. She has published papers describing both ethical problems and psychiatric issues in general medicine.

Anne Hunsaker Hawkins is professor in the Department of Humanities at the Pennsylvania State University College of Medicine. Recent book-length publications include *Reconstructing Illness: Studies in Pathography* (Purdue University Press, 1993, rev. ed., 1999) and *A Small, Good Thing: Stories about Children with HIV and Those Who Care for Them* (W.W. Norton, 2000). She also coedited, with Marilyn McEntyre, *Teaching Literature and Medicine*, a volume in the Modern Language Association's Options for Teaching series (2000).

Anne Hudson Jones is professor of literature and medicine at the Institute for the Medical Humanities of the University of Texas Medical Branch at Galveston, where she teaches courses in literature and medicine and medical humanities. A founding editor of *Literature and Medicine*, she served as the journal's editor in chief for more than a decade. She has published articles on narrative ethics in the *Journal of Medicine and Philosophy, The Lancet, British Medical Journal, HEC Forum*, and the book *Narrative Based Medicine*, (BMJ Books, 1998), which has recently been translated into Japanese. She is coeditor, with Faith McLellan, of the recent book *Ethical Issues in Biomedical Publication* (Johns Hopkins, 2000). In 2000, she became an associate editor of *Annals of Internal Medicine*.

John D. Lantos is associate director of the MacLean Center for Clinical Medical Ethics, director of the Robert Wood Johnson Clinical Scholars Program, and chief of general pediatrics at the University of Chicago. Dr. Lantos has written two books, *Do We Still Need Doctors?* (Routledge,1997) and *The Lazarus Case: Life and Death Issues in Neonatal Intensive Care*, (Johns Hopkins Press, 2001), many papers and book chapters, and is editor (with Carl Elliott) of *The Last Physician: Walker Percy and the Moral Life of Medicine* (Duke, 1999) and (with Roberto Burgio) of *Primum Non Nocere Today* (Elsevier, 1996). He was a member of President Clinton's Health Care Reform Task Force, was president of the American Society of Law, Medicine, and Ethics in 1999, and is on the board of directors of the American Society of Bioethics and Humanities.

Richard Martinez is a physician on the faculty of the Program in Bioethics and Humanities and the Department of Psychiatry at the University of Colorado Health Sciences Center in Denver. After practicing psychiatry for numerous years, he completed a masters of humanities at the University of Colorado, Denver, before going to Harvard University, where he completed fellowships in medical ethics at Harvard Medical School and professional ethics at the Center for Ethics and the Professions in Cambridge. Currently, he directs the ethics curriculum for psychiatric residents, coordinates clinical ethics activities at University of Colorado Hospital, and practices psychotherapy. He has written articles and chapters on medical education, professional ethics, health policy, and physician-writer Walker Percy.

Martha Montello is assistant professor of history and philosophy of medicine, assistant professor of pediatrics, and cochair of the Pediatric Ethics Committee at the University of Kansas School of Medicine. She holds a doctorate in literature from the University of Maryland. Her scholarship focusing on narrative approaches to bioethics and ethical issues in medical education has been published in the *Journal of Clinical Ethics, Annals of Internal Medicine, Academic Medicine, New Orleans Review*, and the *Boston Studies in the Philosophy of Science*. She serves on the editorial boards of *Journal of Medical Humanities* and *Perspectives in Biology and Medicine*.

Kathryn Montgomery is professor of medical ethics and humanities and of medicine at Northwestern University Medical School and director of its Medical Ethics and Humanities Program. She is the author of *Doctors' Stories: The Narrative Structure of Medical Knowledge* (Princeton, 1991) and continues to be almost finished with *Is Medicine a Science? Rationality in an Uncertain Practice*, a study of the formation of clinical judgment.

David B. Morris is a writer and lives in New Mexico. As a scholar of British literature, he wrote many essays and two prize-winning books—*The Religious Sublime* (Kentucky, 1972) and *Alexander Pope: The Genius of Sense* (Harvard, 1984)—before resigning his professorship in 1982 in order to write full-time. His *The Culture of Pain* (University of California, 1991) won a PEN prize. He has subsequently delivered plenary lectures to numerous medical groups, and in 1999 he served as Gunn-Loke Lecturer at the University of Washington Multidisciplinary Pain Center. His most recent books are *Earth Warrior* (Fulcrum, 1995), which describes a voyage he took with environmental activist Paul Watson on an antidriftnet campaign in the North Pacific, and *Illness and Culture in the Postmodern Age* (University of California, 1998).

Hilde Lindemann Nelson is associate professor of philosophy at Michigan State University. A former editor of the *Hastings Center Report*, she is coauthor, with James Lindemann Nelson, of *The Patient in the Family* (Routledge, 1995) and *Alzheimer's: Answers to Hard Questions for Families* (Doubleday, 1997). She has edited two collections, *Feminism and Families* (Routledge, 1997) and *Stories and Their Limits: Narrative Approaches to Bioethics* (Routledge, 1997). She also coedits the *Feminist Constructions* series for Rowman and Littlefield. Her most recent book is *Damaged Identities, Narrative Repair* (Cornell, 2001). Her articles on feminist ethics have appeared in *Hypatia* and a number of edited collections. Her articles in bioethics have appeared in the *Hastings Center Report*, the *Journal of Clinical Ethics*, the *Kennedy Institute of Ethics Journal*, the *Journal of Law, Medicine and Ethics*, and *Bioethics*.

Suzanne Poirier is professor of literature and medical education at the University of Illinois at Chicago College of Medicine, where she has taught students from all branches of the health professions for over twenty years. With her colleague in nursing, Lioness Ayres, she is coauthor of *Stories of Family Caregiving: Reconsiderations of Theory, Literature, and Life*, forthcoming from Sigma Theta Tau Press. She is currently working on a book-length study of physicians' memoirs since 1965.

Walter M. Robinson is assistant professor of pediatrics and social medicine at Harvard Medical School, where he directs the Fellowship in Medical Ethics and teaches ethics to first-year medical students. He is an attending physician in pulmonary medicine and a consultant in ethics and palliative care at Children's Hospital. Dr. Robinson is a faculty scholar in the Project on Death in America and was a senior fellow in the Program in Ethics and the Professions. His research interests include ethical issues in chronic illness and the ethics of pediatric research, and his most recently published works appear in the *Journal of Clinical Ethics*, the *New England Journal of Medicine*, and *Ethics and Behavior*. He is currently working on a social history of cystic fibrosis.

Susan B. Rubin is a philosopher, ethicist, and cofounder of the Ethics Practice, a firm devoted to providing bioethics education, research, and clinical consultation on a national basis. She has served as a consulting ethicist in a variety of acute and long-term care settings, establishing ethics programs, setting up, training, and supporting the ongoing work of ethics committees, and providing ongoing educational and consultation support for health care professionals, institutions, and organizations. Dr. Rubin is author of the book *When Doctors Say No: The Battleground of Medical Futility* (Indiana, 1998) and coeditor of the book *Margin of Error: The Ethics of Mistakes in the Practice of Medicine* (University Publishing Group, 2000) Her articles have appeared in the *Journal of Clinical Ethics*, *Theoretical Medicine, Topics in Stroke Rehabilitation, Health Care Ethics Committee Forum, Modern Healthcare*, and *Healthcare Forum*.

Laurie Zoloth is professor of social ethics and Jewish philosophy and chair of the Jewish studies program at San Francisco State University. She also has worked as a clinical ethicist for fifteen years and served as the president of the American Society for Bioethics and Humanities, the chair of the Howard Hughes Medical Institute Bioethics Advisory Board, and a member of the NASA National Advisory Board. Her book on justice and health care reform, *Health Care and the Ethics of Encounter* (UNC Press, 1999), is a study of Jewish texts and Emmanuel Levinas.

Portions of chapter 3, by Laurie Zoloth and Rita Charon, "Like an Open Book: Reliability, Intersubjectivity, and Textuality in Bioethics," appeared in Laurie Zoloth, "Making the Things of the World: Narrative Construction and the Project of Bioethics," *American Journal of Bioethics* 1, no. 1 (Winter 2001): 59–61.

Portions of Chapter 9, by Charles M. Anderson and Martha Montello, "The Reader's Response and Why It Matters in Biomedical Ethics," appeared in Charles M. Anderson, "Narrative in Biothics," *American Journal of Bioethics* 1, no. 1 (Winter 2001): 61–62.